MUST BE
ON 'ROIDS

MUST BE ON 'ROIDS

A Weight-Training Manual

Mathew James Barnett

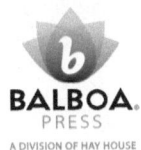

BALBOA.
PRESS
A DIVISION OF HAY HOUSE

Balboa Press books may be ordered through booksellers or by contacting:

Balboa Press
A Division of Hay House
1663 Liberty Drive
Bloomington, IN 47403
www.balboapress.com.au
1-(877) 407-4847

ISBN: 978-1-4525-0919-8 (sc)
ISBN: 978-1-4525-0920-4 (e)

Printed in the United States of America

Balboa Press rev. date: 02/26/2013

CONTENTS

DISCLAIMER

This *book* and information enclosed within it contains restricted and/or privileged information and is intended only for authorized screening and/or confidential presentation at the *said author's* discretion. If you are not the intended observer of this *book*, you must not disseminate, modify, copy/plagiarize or take any action in reliance upon it, unless permitted by the *said author* of the *book*. None of the materials provided on this *book* may be used, reproduced or transmitted, in any form or by any means, electronic or mechanical, including recording or the use of any information storage and retrieval system, without written permission from the *said author*.

If you received this *book* in error, please notify the *said author* immediately.

The confidential nature of and/or privilege in the *book* enclosed is not waived or lost as a result of a mistake or error in this *book*.

The *said author* accepts no liability whatsoever, whether it was caused by:

1. Accessing or other related actions on this *book*.
2. Any links, and/or materials provided/attached to this *book*.

The *said author* assumes that all users understand the risks involved within this *book* and/or its attached materials.

PREFACE

The book came about from my own belief that I have something to offer. People can gain from my experience in weight training. I have something for all levels including beginners to intermediate and advanced bodybuilders.

The name of this book comes from the response I had from other people at the gym. In my home town gym, I have seen two different owners during my membership. One asked my training partner about me and one asked me directly. Saying, "He must be on roids". Hence that became the name for the book.

Another high compliment came from the same gym. We noticed the whole gym was eventually using the same system as us. By watching us train, they changed the way they trained to the way we were training. High praise, as I was not the biggest guy in that gym.

I would like to acknowledge my training partner, Steve, who is my brother. We jointly refined and discovered the best way to train for massive gains and respect.

I would also like to thank YOU, for buying this book. You can trust in knowing that I have poured my heart into this book making sure I left nothing out. While it took a long time, it is worth it.

To your success,
M. J. Barnett.

INTRODUCTION

You are about to take a journey with me, that will take you to a higher standard of bodybuilding. The information here will ask you to push through your current threshold and understand what is meant by 'no pain, no gain'. I make no apology for that corny statement. Go and read the chapter called 'Sheer Guts' to see what you have signed up for.

This book is written for all levels of bodybuilding. Sections have been added to cater for those people who have not been inside a gym before. See the chapter titled 'Beginners Game Plan' and also the exercise descriptions given for each muscle group. The rest of you will have no need to read these descriptions, being familiar with the different exercises.

For the sake of keeping it simple, any reference to a 'rep' will mean the number of repetitions performed for any particular exercise e.g, bench press for 10 reps.

Any reference to a 'set' will mean the number of times an exercise will be performed with rest between each, e.g bench press for 4 sets. Putting it together we get bench press, 4 sets of 10 reps.

So, you do 10 reps, rest a minute, 10 reps again, rest again, 10 reps, rest, 10 reps, you are done. Simple stuff, right!

You will find out what I mean by 'experimenting' and why it is so crucial to getting the most out of the time you spend in the gym, or in a home gym. This idea is experience on a platter for you.

Do you know you have fast and slow muscle fibers? Well you do, and they require different approaches to enable you to stimulate their growth. I want you to know the 'why' as well as the 'how'.

Sheer guts; a key chapter in this book. I talk about how I train. I also tell you what I think is your secret weapon, for massive gains in size, definition, strength and power.

Spotting each other; if I had to pick one chapter that tells my story, this is it. I am not kidding when I say; the whole gym adopted my approach to spotting. They looked at me, saw how I trained and copied it. I am going to make you laugh too, in this chapter. A quick story about spotting I once saw.

As you can see in the contents, there is a lot in this book. I am keeping it as short as I can. But, I need to cover everything I do, which you will be able to copy.

Let me tell you this, my new friend. I am more excited about getting your feedback on your gains than actually selling this book.

Every single message is going to get me buzzing with pride. Your feedback and questions can be sent to the email I set up for this book; see the last page. If I keep getting the same types of questions from people, I will link this email to a Blog site. That will also allow readers to see questions by others.

THE EXPERIMENT

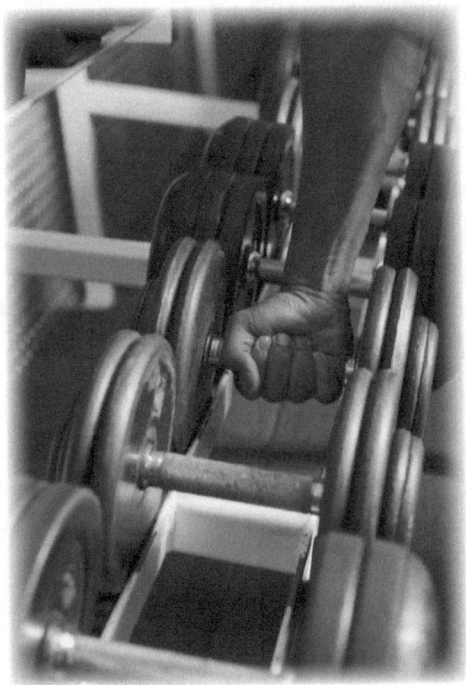

Before you get into your bodybuilding program, you have to take some time in the gym, to do some experimenting. While this is very easy to do, it will take a few trips to the gym. You will be asked to do exercises with low reps and high reps.

We will use bench press as an example. You will do strength sets and cutting sets, or definition sets. Strength sets will be low reps, say around 6 to 8 reps while cutting sets will be high rep, say around 10 to 12 reps or more.

So off you go and do bench press. After a warm up or light set to get the blood flowing, you do 2 sets of 6 reps and another 2 sets of 12 reps on the bench press. You think you did it right, because that's what I said you should do. Not quite!

Whatever level you are at, there will be a weight for every exercise you do that is just right for you. By experimenting, you will find it. Using bench press as our example again, I am looking for my 6 rep weight. I will warm up again, with one or two light sets.

Then I try different weights until I find that I can just get the 6th rep out. The last rep, the 6th, will be slow and you might strain a little.

Rest and repeat once. You will get 4, 5, or 6 reps out the second time. That's great. I will explain more on this later. You will keep that weight until you get 2 sets out of 8 however how long that takes, weeks, months etc. Then you will increase the weight and do 6's again, until you get to 2 sets of 8. Repeat, repeat, repeat. Note that bench press is by far the most effective exercise for your chest.

After warming up, I prefer 3 or 4 sets of 6 to 8 reps and then do the 10 to 12 reps by 2 or 3 sets. It's really two exercises on the one piece of equipment, one for bulking and one for cutting up.

The 12 rep bench press weight is found the same way. You will warm up with one or two sets and then experiment with weights until you find your weight. You will breathe heavily and stain a little for the last two reps. Rest and repeat. This time you may get only 10 reps out as you are now fatigued. Fantastic so far. You will get to two sets of 12 reps after some time, weeks or months.

As your 6 rep weights go up, so will the 12 rep weights. Even start at 2 sets of 10 reps and work up to 12 reps.

When you are doing bench press in your workout after you know which weights to use, you will do two warm up sets first. They will be 8 to 10 reps each and the second set must be heavier than the first. Then you will do the 6 rep sets, followed by the 12 rep sets; more on this later.

You should have a training partner with you. They are not allowed to touch the weight. They are your safety guys only. That is, if you're done, and the weight is sitting on your chest, or you are stuck and can't push any more, they will help you put it back on the rack; but only after you tell them. Nothing worse than an eager spotter taking it off you too soon. The reason for this training partner method will be explained in a later chapter. Let's do some more examples on different muscles.

BICEPS: We will be doing seated dumbbell curls. You will curl one arm at a time.

You want an 8 rep weight for this. If you can do 10 or 12 or more reps, the weight is too light. You want some strain on the last one or two reps. A little burn on this last one or two reps is your goal. As with all exercises, you will do one or two warm up sets with a lighter weight. Warm up sets do not count.

You must do 3 sets, after the warm up sets, I prefer 4, but you decide. Your sets might be 8 reps, 8 reps, 7 reps and 6 reps. That is fine. You will get to a point where you feel like doing 10 reps each set, just to feel the burn that you felt when you started with that weight. Well you guessed it. It's time to increase the weight again. It's that simple. Repeat, repeat, repeat.

You will do three exercises on biceps, which will be explained later. For example, you will do the seated or standing, if you prefer, dumbbell curls (4 by 8 reps). You will do standing barbell curls (4 by 8 reps). You will also do what I call concentration curls (4 by 12 reps), which I will explain in full details later.

SHOULDERS: We will start with seated barbell press. All gyms have a chair with the rack attached for you to pick the bar up from behind your head. You are looking for your 8 rep weight here. You must feel the strain and burn on the 8th rep, or it's too light for you. You will do 3 or 4 sets here as well. You might start doing 8 reps, 8 reps, 7 reps, and 6 reps; Fantastic. When you need to do all sets of 9 or 10 to get your burn, you are ready to increase the weight.

Don't forget your warm up sets here too. As with all exercises, they are not part of the 3 or 4 sets you are doing, they are extra's. I will be talking more on warming up later.

You will do three or four exercises on shoulders. You must work all three deltoids, front, side and rear. I will give you the reps and you will do the experiment.

You could do behind neck barbell press (4 by 8 rep); seated dumbbell press (4 by 8 rep); upright row (4 by 10-12 rep), and bent side laterals (4 by 8 reps). I will be giving a full description of the exercises later.

You will be able to find your weight for any exercise on any muscle group now. If I stopped writing here, you would have enough to make massive gains.

The experiments are that crucial, allowing your time in the gym to be the most productive. I didn't get asked if I was on steroids just from experimenting, so keep reading.

Now that you're aware of this, you will see people go into a gym and pick up any old weight and start repping away.

They think that they must be right, just because they are doing the exercise the same way everyone else does it. It's good to watch others in the gym for pointers, but take no notice of how much weight they use. You know exactly how to find what weights you must use now! You now have my first key to effective bodybuilding.

HIT BOTH MUSCLE FIBER TYPES

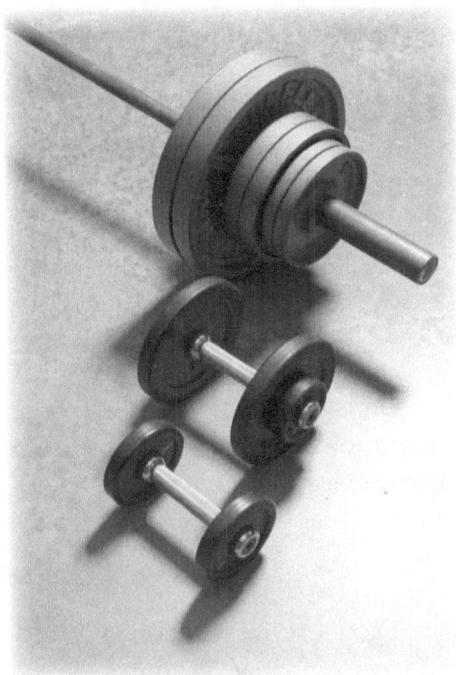

The first one is your abs. You won't get a burn after doing 8 crunches, or inclined sit-ups, or leg raises, or standing pulley crunches. You will need many more reps per set. Some of you will need to do sets of 50 before you get any burning feeling, where it starts to get harder and causes you to strain. I like to mix my abb workouts up. There is enough equipment for you to change your exercises around as you like. If your gym has six pieces of equipment, you can use them.

Everyone's muscles are made up of fast and slow twitching fibers. Because of this, you will need to train so that you are using both fiber types. When you are training a muscle, you must do some high rep sets and some low rep sets. There are two ways to do this. Firstly, you could do more sets, some high reps and some low reps, for any particular exercise. I mentioned earlier that I like to do this with bench press.

You could also mix the combination of exercises you do for a muscle group.

Take biceps as our example. I will do heavy dumbbell curls, for 8 reps each set. After warm up, I suggest three or four sets, where you aim for 8 reps; then do barbell curls.

You can do high reps here as an option. Try three or four sets of 12 reps. I like a fairly heavy weight, and a target of 10 reps for the four sets.

Finish off with some concentration curls (I will explain the exercises in a later chapter) where you do 12 reps with a suitable lighter weight. Again I like three or four sets aiming for the 12 reps each time.

On all of these sets, you may only get your target reps done on the first two sets. Then achieve a lower rep count on the next set or two. That's fine. With the example on biceps, we have done heavy, lower rep sets for your fast fibers and the lighter weight for high rep sets hitting the slow fibers.

You can see then that if you just did one type of exercise, either high rep lighter weights, or the low rep heavy weights, you would not achieve a complete expansion of all the muscle fibers in your body.

For those of you that might need to explain this to someone else, I will try to give a better definition. Every muscle has three parts, with exception of fat and water. There are slow twitching red fibers and fast twitching white fibers, plus the blood capillaries. Heavy training such as powerlifting, builds mostly fast twitching fibers which leaves the slow twitching fibers undeveloped.

You can see that athletes in shot-put, discus and powerlifting are very strong. But, they will not have the definition in their muscles as someone who train's as a bodybuilder.

The workout programs in the back of this book address the need to train both fiber types. I have always done my workouts with a mix of low rep and high rep sets for every muscle I train.

But, I want to add to that by saying that there are exceptions to the rule. There are two muscle groups that seem to ignore this fast and slow fiber rule.

The first muscle is your abbs. These muscles will not respond to sets of low reps, like 3 sets of 12 reps. The three sets will more likely have to be 30, 40 or 50 reps per set.

You will be given more exercises than you need for your abbs. The benefit of that is so you can mix it up a little.

The second muscle is your calves. My magic number on calves is 25 reps. I like to do sitting calve raises, standing calve raises and toe press on the incline leg-press machine. Take a wild guess, and that's all it is, but I would imagine that these muscles may have more slow twitching fibers than fast fibers. Who knows? Is it important? No its not, you only want to really know how to train the muscle. I could look it up and make a big deal of it, but the book is about what to do in the gym for massive growth and definition.

I did mention earlier that I will explain the why and the how. But only if it fits in with the flow. I want to get you to the end of this book as quickly as possible, with only crucial information, and no wasted reading. So let's keep going.

My message here is that I will be putting the sets and reps that I do for each exercise in the workouts towards the back. You will see low rep and high rep sets. Why? So that I can hit both types of fibers.

So I had to include this chapter to let you know that you can't miss any parts in the workouts I give you. Sure, you can mix it up, but you still have to do some low reps and some high reps for each muscle. I knew there was a reason for the why of it all. You now have my next key to efficient bodybuilding.

Before you read on, let's just look at the ways I mix it up, using biceps as our example again. I will use three examples of doing different sets and reps with three different exercises. Dumbbell curls, barbell curls and restricted or what I call concentration curls (again, these will be described later in this book).

1ST EXAMPLE	2ND EXAMPLE	3RD EXAMPLE
Dumbbells 4 lots of 8 reps	Dumbbells 4 lots of 12 reps	Dumbbells 4 lots of 8 reps
Barbell 4 lots of 8 reps	Barbell 4 lots of 8 reps	Barbell 4 lots of 12 reps
Concentration 4 by 12 reps	Concentration 4 by 12 reps	Concentration 4 by 12 reps

Now, you are probably thinking; that's great Mat, but when do I use the different mixes? Thank you for asking that question. I like to do the first example for the majority of the time.

This means that I will do it for three months and then do a month of the second or third example. Actually, during that month, I do the second example for a week, then the third example for a week, and so on, for one month, or a little more.

COMPOUND EXERCISES

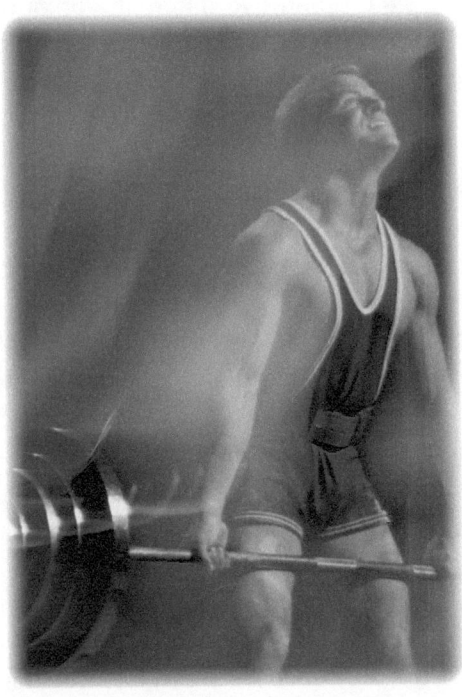

Compound exercises use several different muscles at the same time. These are the exercises where you will handle the heaviest loads in your workout routines. Some compound exercises include bench press, deadlifts, squats and incline leg press. These exercises will also help grow other muscle groups that are not directly used during the movement. I personally noticed a marked increase in overall strength after I made an effort to go harder on my deadlifts. The heavy weights involved seem to give stimulation to the other muscles, all over your body. You won't see many people doing these harder exercises, such as deadlifts.

You will have a more productive workout if you do your compound exercises toward the beginning of your workout. Using the heavier weights makes them much more taxing on your energy levels. The next thing you can do is to split the compound exercises into different workouts, where possible. I use the compound exercises to dictate the muscles that I will train on any given day.

Bench press uses your chest muscle primarily. I'm sure you know that, but some don't. The other muscle is your triceps, at the back of your arm, behind your biceps. Without fail, I always do chest and triceps on the same day only if I am doing two different workouts per week, which I prefer. You will add other muscle groups, doing a total of four muscle groups each workout / day. So I do legs, chest, triceps and abbs on one day of the two day split routine.

You will be wondering why I train legs with chest, as both are categorized as having compound exercises in the routine. It is mainly a process of elimination. Or, more of what compound exercises you don't want to do on the same workout / day. I find that my legs workout is not detrimental to my chest workout. But my back workout which includes deadlifts is detrimental to my chest workout. I also train chest and shoulders on different days.

My back workout also stimulates my shoulders. So there are two more muscle groups that I must train on the same workout / day; back and shoulders. On a two days split routine, I do back, shoulders, biceps and forearms.

I just want to confirm the two days split routine concept. You have two different workouts, so you are splitting the body's muscles into two workouts. You might train each workout twice per week, for a total of four workouts for the week. Or do each workout three times, for a total of six for the week.

I have included this section on compound exercises so that you will know why I train certain muscles together and don't vary from it. The compound exercises, bench press, squats and deadlifts tell you what muscles compliment each other. You will have few injuries as well. How? Muscles need time off, which is when they are growing.

If your workouts continually stimulate a particular muscle, it is continually broken down and growth will be restricted. Injuries will be very likely under these conditions.

Your job is to train every muscle group. You want maximum results for your effort. This means hitting the muscle group today and letting it rest tomorrow before hitting it again the next day.

By understanding the effect compound exercises, you won't over train your muscles and risk injury. You will also give them time to rest and grow.

If you are short on time and still want to hit the gym for a quick workout. You will get the most out of your limited time if you just do compound exercises. Why? Because compound exercises increase your metabolism and testosterone levels. This gives you quicker muscle growth. You will be stimulating more than one muscle with every exercise, so there is a good level of efficiency there too. You would be hard pressed to find someone who suggests doing isolation exercises instead of compound exercises.

Compound exercises are the perfect starting point for those of you who have not done bodybuilding before, or have had a very long spell between sessions. This type of workout will be covered later in this book.

COMPOUND EXERCISES AND MUSCLES THEY STIMULATE:

Primary muscle (P) and other muscles (O) that are affected by the compound movement.

EXERCISE	Muscle (P)	Muscle (O)	Muscle (O)	Muscle (O)
Deadlift's	Back	Shoulder's	Bicep's	Forearm's
Bench Press	Chest	Triceps		
Squat's	Leg (thigh)	Leg (quads)	Leg (hamstring)	Lower back
Behind Neck Press	Shoulder's	Bicep's		
Stiff Leg Deadlift	Leg (hamstring)	Lower Back		
Chinup's	Back (lats)	Back (traps)	Shoulder's	Bicep's

There's a full body workout right there, based on doing only compound movements. Someone coming back after a layoff or just starting out can do this combination for two or three months, twice to three times per week. I will show some more compound exercises but above are the main ones. There's a whole chapter on this, keep reading!

ISOLATION EXERCISES

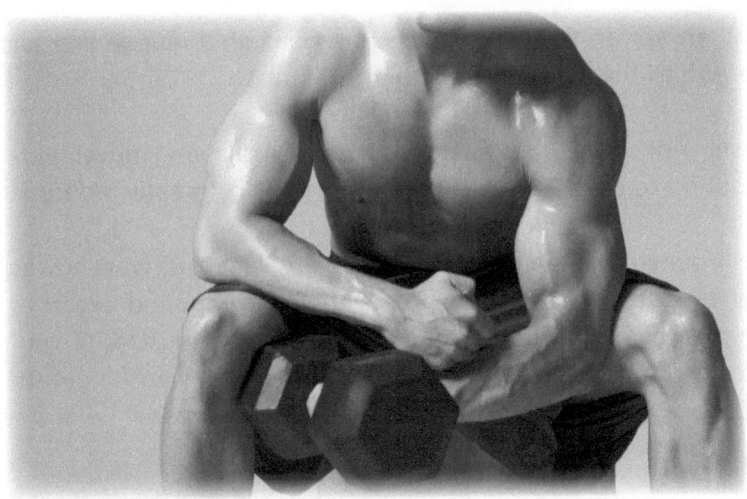

These exercises work one muscle group. They allow you to focus on just one body part. Isolation exercises compliment your compound exercises. With the compound exercises, some muscles only get indirect stimulation. For proper growth, you need to work each muscle directly. You therefore need isolation exercises in your workout routine. To clarify that point, a beginner does not 'need' isolation exercises.

An example of 'one muscle group' is biceps. Doing dumbbell curls will focus directly on your biceps, making them an isolation exercise. Your muscle definition or the 'ripple effect' will come from your work on isolation exercises. As a bodybuilder, they are simply vital.

You will lift the heavier weights in your workout during the compound exercises. But, you will also feel the pain doing the isolation aspect of your workouts. This direct focus will give you a 'pump' provided you can withstand the pain long enough. This focusing aspect will be covered in the next chapter. Read on!

As you move through your workout, you will exhaust your muscles one at a time. Even using lighter weights, you will find your isolation exercises particularly intense. The order in which you train your muscles is vital.

You will always do the compound movement on a muscle first and then follow with all the isolation movements.

You will not have the energy to train isolation movements then compound exercises. The level of efficiency will be greatly reduced.

You will generally train your larger muscles first and work towards the smaller muscles last. Combine this with the compound exercises done first and follow with your isolation exercise, on all muscles. If you follow this, you will be able to hit each muscle harder. You want to get the most out of every workout, so all of my workout programs will be in a specific order.

A quick word on which comes first; compound or isolation movements (exercises). There are advocates of doing the isolation exercises before the compound exercises.

Let us use chest as an example with the isolation exercises first. We will do incline fly's with light dumbbells followed by the peck-deck machine.

Then do dumbbell pullovers with a moderate sized dumbbell. Last, we do bench-press which requires the heaviest weight out of the four exercises.

Do you think after the first three exercises, where you have really pushed yourself? You will be able to do a good bench press? My answer is no way. How will you handle the heavy compound exercise (bench-press) when you have exhausted your muscles on the lighter weights.

I know it is much better to do the heavier lifts early for each body part. You will still fatigue the muscle after the bench press, but you will be able to handle the lighter weights during the rest of the exercises. You will still be able to achieve a burn and push through that burn for a few more reps. That is in the next chapter, so more later.

My last point is that it is safer. In what way, you ask. With my method of training, I can go to the gym by myself and still use the same weights. You will know what you can lift and how far past your burning reps you can go. You will lift the maximum efficient weight for every exercise on each body part. This is all part of my routine which led to people asking if I was on roids, which has now led to this book. If my results were not so great, I would have nothing to write about. But I do and you are reading it. I also want to hear about your experience with my method. Anyway, back on track.

I want to show you how I put my compound exercises with my isolation exercises. So, I'll start with each body part and list the exercises in my bag of tricks.

I will also mark them as (/comp) for compound and (/isol) for isolation. The exercises will be explained later in the book. For now I just want to list them.

LEGS:

LEGS	Squatts / comp	Incline Press / comp
Leg extension / isol	Leg curl / isol	Stiff Leg Deadlift / isol
Standing calves / isol	Seated calves / isol	Toe press / isol

You will be doing all of these exercises in your leg workouts; eight in total.

CHEST:

CHEST	Bench press / comp	Incline Dumbbell / comp
Incline barbell / comp	Dips / isol	Pullovers / isol
Peck-Deck / isol	Incline fly / isol	Cable Crossover / isol

Do the compound exercises first, ranked by weight used, so bench press is always first. You will pick four exercises from this list, bench press plus three more.

You will mix them up, and use them all over a short period of time. The (*) shows that it is the same exercise; you will do one or the other.

TRICEPS:

TRICEP	Z-Bar press / isol	Close-grip bench / isol
Dumbbell dips / isol	1 Arm tricep press / isol	Lat machine press / isol
Dumbbell kickback / isol *		

Pick three or four for each workout. I like the variety, plus it keeps your muscles from getting used to one exercise. Otherwise, your muscles get a bit stale and don't grow as well. Keep shocking your muscles with variety. Don't underestimate this point.

ABS:

ABS	Incline situp / isol	hanging leg raise / isol
Bench leg raise / isol	Pulley crunch / isol	Barbell twist / isol
Crunch / isol	Knee ups / isol	

Pick three or four and then swap around after a week or two. You might be wondering about the sets and reps that you should be doing. I will include that in the workouts I have put towards the back of this book. You will also get the full description for each exercise in another section later on.

On a two day split routine, these are the four body parts I train in one session at the gym. You can see that a bodybuilder has far more isolation exercises in their bag of tricks than compound exercises. The two day split routine means that you divide the body parts into two workouts. I like training on Monday, Tuesday, Thursday and Friday, for example.

I usually do each workout twice in a week. We will cover more of these later in the book. I will show you my four, five and six days per week routines.

The other workout routine in the two day split routine includes shoulders, back, biceps and forearms. So between the two workouts, you will cover your whole body. Let's have a look at the exercises now!

SHOULDERS:

SHOULDER	B.N.Press / comp	Military press / comp
Dumbbell press / comp	Upright row / comp	Bent side lats / isol
Side laterals / comp		

Your shoulder muscles have three lobes or heads. Front lobe, side lobe and rear lobe.

The compound exercises work all the three lobes, but mostly the front lobes. For this reason, I do extra isolation movements for the side and rear lobes. (*) Shows that they are the same exercise; just pick one per workout. You must do all five exercises.

The thing to remember here is to do the compound exercises before the isolation exercises.

The workouts I give in the back are in set order. So don't be concerned about the order of exercises.

BACK:

BACK	Deadlift / comp	Chinups / comp
Lat pulldown / isol	Pulley row / isol	bent row / isol
Shrugs / isol	Stiff leg deadlift / isol	1 Arm row / isol

I will talk more on this later, but a strong back is crucial to being successful in bodybuilding. Correct form or technique while training your back is vital. Some of these isolation exercises are done with quite heavy weights.

If you are standing while bent over or sitting and doing back exercises, you must keep your chin up. It helps keep your back straight. The first time you arch your back under strain from an exercise, you can easily pull a muscle in your back.

You will do deadlifts and chinups plus any three exercises you like. I like to rotate every week or two, between the isolation exercises. This means you will do five exercises for every back workout. I will explain why, later, but I do chin-ups last, all the time. Let's move right along!

BICEPS:

BICEP	Dumbbell curl / isol	Barbell curl / isol
Z-Bar curl / isol	Preacher curl / isol	Concentration curl / isol
Pulley curl / isol		

(*) and (**) show that the exercises are basically the same and you can pick one or the other. You can do four bicep isolation movements in each workout, but no less than three. For a week or two, you can do concentration curls, then swap for preacher curls. I like dumbbell curls and barbell curls or preacher curls, plus one or two more isolation exercises. When I'm in the gym, if there is a Z-Bar not being used, I prefer it, because it's more comfortable on your wrists. Otherwise, you can just use the straight bars for barbell curls. Notice that all of the exercises are isolation movements.

While your biceps are stimulated from the compound movements done for other body parts, your biceps need the direct stimulus the isolation exercise give.

FOREARM:

FOREARM	Wrist curl / isol	Reverse curl / isol
Grip machine / isol	Reverse wrist curl / isol	

All the forearm exercises are isolation movements. After you finish doing biceps, your forearms will already be stimulated. You will not need many sets to get that burning sensation.

So there is my arsenal of exercises for each body part. You can see I prefer free weights over machines. I have a chapter on the reasons for that later in the book. I hope I have explained sufficiently that you need compound and isolation exercises as a bodybuilder.

The next chapter is another key chapter, on what it takes to look like a bodybuilder

SHEER GUTS

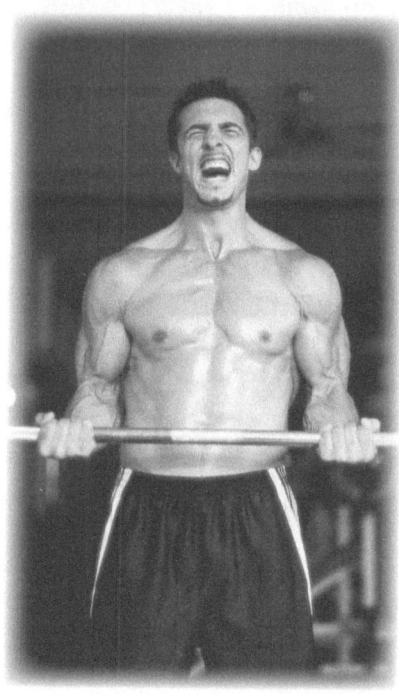

Consider this! You're at the gym and you spot someone who has a rippling hard body. It's obvious to you their results are from total dedication. Maybe you have even thought to yourself, he must be on roids. Yah, me too.

But have you ever wondered just what it takes to actually look like a bodybuilder. I remember for example, thinking that it is as easy as monkey see monkey do. All I have to do is watch what "they" do and copy, right!

Yes (1) and No (2):

1. Yes, because you want to adopt the correct technique for every exercise. With correct techniques, comes efficiency. By that I mean you get the most out of every single workout. What? Strict form and technique is much harder to perform than just sloppy movements with least pain and resistance. So which path will you follow? The one with least resistance or the one with much of it to maximize your time in the gym.
2. No, because you must use weights for your size and strength, not what some bodybuilder has worked up to. And no because you can't be sure that the person you watch knows how to train hard and efficiently. What? They might have a nice big rippling body but what if their system took eight years to achieve. Can you wait that long?

So what does it take then? Sheer guts. Let me explain. If you haven't already felt the burn from pumping iron, soon you will by following this. It's how you respond to that very uncomfortable sensation that really matters.

In my opinion, it seems that vast majority of people will quit the movement as soon as they feel discomfort. Let me just get it out there now. That is not what I do.

You need to know that it's vital for you to push through the discomfort of the burn. By that, I mean you must keep going, and do one, two, three or four more reps in that set you are on.

You also need to know that in doing so, you get instant reward. Pushing through the pain releases endorphins which are a mild high.

After your workout, you will be tired and fatigued but totally satisfied and exhilarated by the endorphins.

There is even more gratification from the muscle pump you get. Your muscles become bigger and harder than before you started your workout. The truth is that your level of gratification increases with your ability to do these burning reps.

Let me give an example; using bicep dumbbell curls in a seated position. I know what weight will give me a burn after 6 reps, so I do 8 to 10 for best results.

I get a burn from the 6th rep through to the 8th or 10th rep, if I do that many. The four sets after warm-up might go like this; 10 reps, 10 reps, 9 reps and 8 reps.

Pushing through the pain of the burn gives you the knowledge that you are doing your job right. And that is to train to your maximum every set you do. Why? Because it will make you grow at light speed.

We have all heard of the saying; you only get out of it what you put into it. If that didn't originate from some bodybuilder somewhere, it sure could have.

I want you to know that I think this chapter is the most important one in the book. You need to know what is required to get massive muscle growth. And that is, as I see it, sheer guts. In later chapters, I expand on this, giving you more exact insight on a muscle by muscle basis. Just know now that a certain level of mental toughness is required of you.

Even if you feel you may lack in this area, don't worry my friend. If you can follow my instructions, you will end up with a massive rippling physique. And guess what? Your mental toughness will grow with you. That's a win win situation for you.

SPOTTING EACH OTHER

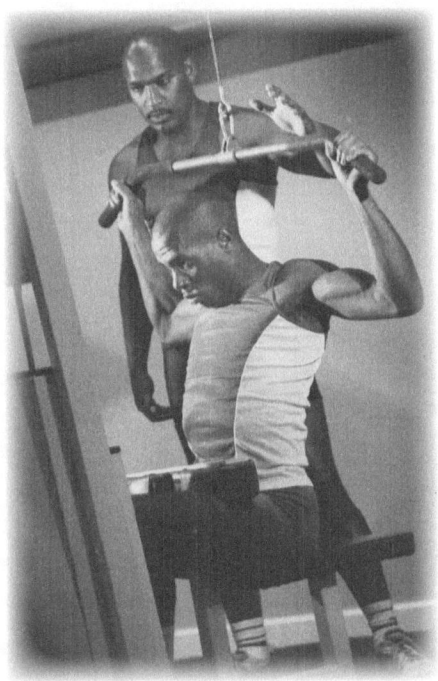

I want to share a short story with you. While it's funny, there's also a message in it. There was a guy who I would see in the gym quite often. He always turned up with his training partner, who was a lot lighter.

On this one occasion, they were doing behind neck press as part of their shoulder workout. Using the gym equipment, one sits on the chair and pushes a barbell above their head, up and down. While their training partners stand on a platform behind them and can easily spot or help replace the barbell after finishing.

When it was the larger guy's turn, I noticed that he put a lot of weight on the bar. It was enough weight for me to think, I got to watch this guy.

He took position on the seat and his spotter stood on the platform behind. He grabs the bar and tries to lift it off the rack and push it up behind his head.

It doesn't budge; he's put too much weight on. He quickly takes some off, still leaving way more than I thought he could handle.

"Help me get it up", he says to his partner. So together, they lift this weighted barbell off the rack. The spotter helps lift the bar until his mate can straighten his arms above his head. OK, spot me for 10. I can't take my eyes off these two guys.

I watch them both strain for eight reps. The spotter doing as much if not most of the work. In defiance, the seated guy yells out "two more". Then comes the comment from the spotter. "I can't do any more".

Did I just hear right? The spotter just said to the guy that's supposed to be doing the movement that he can't do any more. I had to stuff my gym towel in my mouth, so they wouldn't hear me laughing. What a comment. I lost all focus after that and could hardly finish my workout.

So what is the message here? Sometimes learning what not to do is just as important as learning what to do. This story shows what you should not do.

In fact, it seems 100% opposite to what I do. I think that's why I found it so 'fall on the floor' funny.

Let's keep going. This chapter on its own will take you to massive gains. The whole idea of spotting means being able to train to complete muscle fatigue without the risk of dropping the weight on yourself.

Let me give you an example using bench press. From the start, I do a warm-up set and another one with more weight. No spotting just yet. I'm looking for 3 or 4 sets here and warm-ups don't count.

The target is 10 to 12 reps for both warm-up sets. With the 3 or 4 counted sets, the weight will increase. The first counted set will be 8 to 12 reps and no spotting yet. The second set can be much the same i.e. 8 to 12 reps.

What you are doing is setting yourself up to peak at the 3rd and 4th sets. The 3rd set may range from 6 to 10 reps. Your spotter will only help you put the bar back on the bench press rack if you say so.

You might get 7 reps and lower the bar down to your chest for another push; if you start pushing and it seems to be stuck half way up. The spotter must still wait for your call. Why do that? You will develop deep tissue strength.

Sometimes the bar will go up as if in slow motion. But doing it yourself makes all the difference. The 3rd set is at your maximum weight. When you feel ready, you will do a 4th set, which is also at your maximum weight.

The spotter does not help you do more reps, ever. Your spotter is your safety guy or girl. Giving you piece of mind that you can train to fatigue without risk of injury.

The whole gym adopted my approach to spotting. After watching my progress explode, other trainers slowly adopted my method. It took a while as I know old habits die hard; especially when ego comes into it. Anyway, let's keep going.

First I noticed only one or two spotting like I did. Then a few more, until eventually everyone did it. Even the roid brigade copied me.

They obviously saw what it was doing for myself, and wanted the same results for themselves.

I am very open and happy to help. So many took advantage of that and I happily answered many questions. Like, why do you do that? My answer was simple for that particular question; it gives me the fastest gains possible.

It will give you the same; deep tissue growth which provides true power. To me true power is the proportionate increase in strength as my muscles increase in size far from what you get with steroids, but I will cover that next.

One more example though, before we move on. Using seated dumbbell shoulder press. I like a good seat with high support for my back and neck. I also like to sit upright and not be leaning back.

The first set is just a warm-up. By that I mean, using a medium weight. Spotting for this exercise will again only take place at my call, never before. It is up to me to know which weight to use. Your own experiments take care of that for you. You should have it written down until you come to know the weights you need.

So, I want to be fatigued by the 10th rep on each set. 3 or 4 sets will do.

And again, the warm up sets are not counted as part of the 3 or 4 sets, ever. As the weights get heavier, the spotter's job changes for this exercise.

There is a point where the two dumbbells become too heavy to lift off the floor into position, at the same time. Your spotter will load you up, one dumbbell at a time. All the pushing during the set is done by you with no help from the spotter, ever. The spotter stands behind as a safety guard.

Another way you will load up with heavy dumbbells is to stand the dumbbells upright on your knees as you sit down while holding the hand grip of course. Then one at a time, flick your knee up, giving the dumbbell a helping hand, and hold it just above your shoulder. When you have both dumbbells, push up for your first rep.

Unloading can also be done using your knees. By bringing one knee up at a time, stand the dumbbell up on it and do the other dumbbell the same way.

Then stand up and lower the dumbbells to their rack or the floor, with a straight back and head up. Let's keep going.

At the point of failure, you may have got it up half way and felt you can do no more. There is absolutely no point in the spotter taking the strain and helping you push out a few more. Your spotter needs discipline not to jump in without your call.

They should give your deep muscle tissue a chance. As you grow, you will move past these sticking points. As if in slow motion, you will have the power to finish a rep that seemed totally stuck. Spotting the old way will never get you here, ever, ever, ever.

My approach to spotting will get you powerful and massive. And it will happen in record time. As it happened to me, it will happen for you too. PEOPLE WILL THINK YOU MUST BE ON ROIDS!!!!

HE MUST BE ON ROIDS

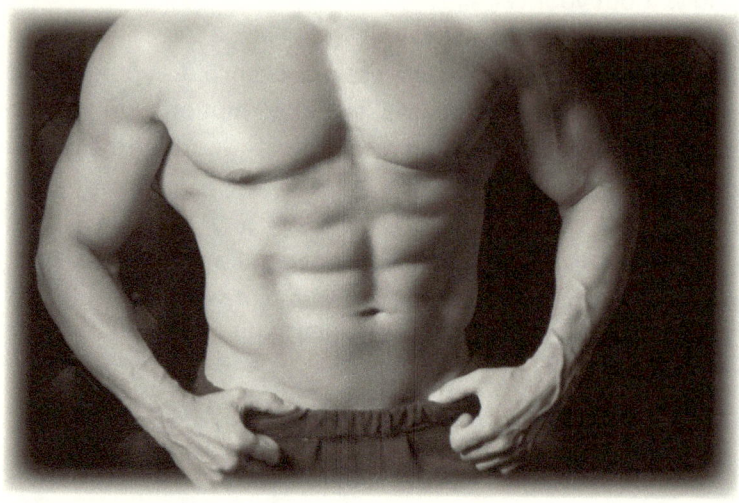

Just for the record, I have never taken steroids. On top of that, I don't see the point. To me, the risks far outweigh the rewards.

While other illegal drugs release dopamine giving you high steroids (anabolic androgenic steroids), they travel the same pathway in your brain, without giving you a high. But they also do the same damage to your brain. The short story is that steroids can cause significant changes in your mood and behavior, much like illegal drugs.

Medical research backs the possibility of psychiatric disorders. Some of these include aggression, paranoid, jealousy, delusions, impaired judgment and violence. Do you need more proof? Ok, here's more.

There are some permanent conditions that steroid users get. How would you like to turn yellow, from jaundice? You may also get high blood pressure, severe liver damage or severe scaring from acne.

Boys, you can lose size in your testicles and have a reduced sperm count. What about baldness or developing breasts. That's not all; you'll get an increased risk of prostate cancer.

Girls, you can develop a deep voice or any or all of these; baldness, facial hair, irregular menstrual cycle or an increase in the size of your clitoris.

Injecting steroids can give you hepatitis or AIDS.

The first time I became aware that people thought I could be on steroids was at my local gym. The owner made a comment to my training partner. I remember being surprised. I was happy with the weights I was using but I never thought I had enough size for people to think I was on roids.

In a strange way it was cool. I knew I wasn't using them, but here's people comparing my size to people who do use roids.

The truth is, I was training hard but I wasn't doing the things I discovered later on. The best was yet to come. By then, there was a new owner of my local gym.

It happened again, the new owner came over to ask me straight out. No way, I explained, not me pal. The thing is, I always thought he was on roids. Him and quite a few others who trained here.

They kind of stood out, at least to me, they did. A group who seemed to love light weights but were all puffed up with veins popping and rippling muscles. But, they were all show and no go.

I spotted for most of them at one time or another. Only ever once for each of them though. It was too much for them. When it got harder, they were used to their partners helping them move the weight. Well, I don't train that way. Many people held on tight to the old way. Call it pride or ego, whatever. Even with proof that spotting isn't the best way in front of their eyes, so many were slow to come around.

I mentioned it earlier, but I'll try to be more specific. The name of this book came about from people thinking I was on roids. Having my gains noticed made me realize I was making good progress in the gym.

Here I am doing some things totally different from everyone in there. In full view and open to all criticism. But as it turned out, I began using some big weights with good form. There was only one result and that was that I got big. And it happened too fast.

So I know I will have the right to pass this on to YOU. That's why I wrote this book. You'll see for yourself. After using my methods, people will make comments and will copy you. When that happens, will you let me know? You'll have done the hard work, but I'll feel like it was all the more worth it to write the book, just to hear it's worked for you as it has for me.

HOW MANY SETS AND HOW MANY REPS?

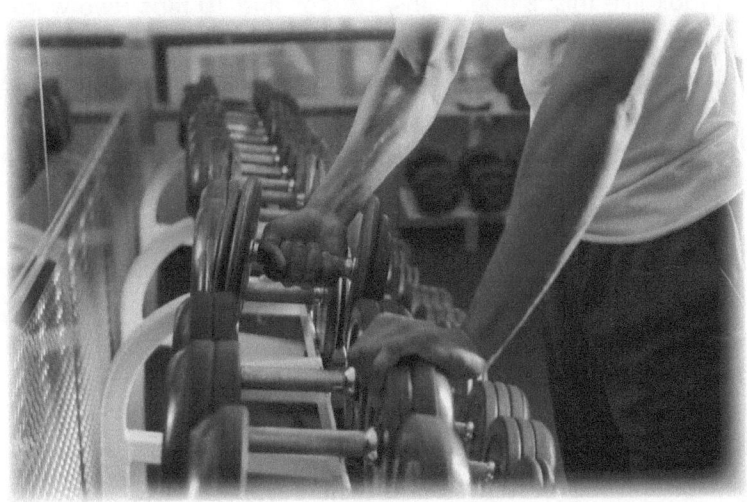

Without exceptions, I do warm-up exercises before I do the counted ones. The warm-up repetitions will always be at the higher end of the scale i.e, 10 or 12 or more.

Take bench press for example. You want to do 12 repetitions with a weight you can handle quite comfortably for your first warm-up set. Then, increase the weight only a little and do another warm-up set, of 10 or 12 reps. That's your warm-up done. Your blood is flowing and your muscles are ready for more!

If you always do warm-up sets, you will have few injuries. The last thing you want is a strain or a pulled muscle that interferes with your progress.

You won't always have to do two warm-up sets; only if you are starting on a particular muscle. For example, take biceps exercises.

You can do three different exercises in your workout for biceps. They could be barbell curl, dumbbell curl and restricted curl or any three you like.

Whichever exercise you start with, for that muscle, you do the warm-up sets first. For the second and third exercises, your biceps are already warm and you don't need to do a warm-up set for those exercises.

It would look like this: Barbell curls, 12 reps and 10 reps (two warm-ups), then say 10 reps, 8 reps and 8 reps. A total of five sets including the warm-up sets. Dumbbell curls, 10, 8 and 8 reps for a total of three sets.

Restricted curls, 10, 8 and 8 reps for a total of three sets again. That's a total of 11 sets on biceps from the three different exercises.

Now, there are some exceptions to this rule. Some muscle groups have more than one part. Legs have four groups i.e, quads, hamstrings, glutes and calf muscles. Back has lats, traps, upper and lower muscles. Shoulders have front, side and rear deltoid muscles.

When you train these muscles, you can do a warm-up set before each exercise, except the very first one, where you do two warm-up sets. Simple enough!

The number of counted sets, that is the ones after the warm-up sets, will vary. If I'm coming back from a break, I will do two counted sets for a month. If you're just staring out, you'll do the same, but for three months.

The best number of sets will always be 3 or 4, for each exercise. So if you do three exercises per muscle, that's 9 to 12 sets for that muscle.

The best number of repetitions will always be 8. That means, if you start your biceps exercise with heavy dumbbell curls, you might do 8 reps, then another 8 reps, then do 6 reps on the third set. That's very good. There's room to improve the 6 to 8 and you will still grow doing 6.

The first time you sit down and do three sets of 10 reps or 12, 10, 10 or something similar to the above 10 reps, its time to increase your weight and go back to 8 reps.

There are exceptions to these rules. One of those is chin ups. When you are starting out, chinups are very hard. While that is true, you still need to do them. If you normally aim for 3 sets of 8 repetitions, that's 24 reps in total, with that in mind.

If you can only do 3 chinups in one go before you let go, guess how many sets I want you to do? If you said 8, that's right. I want 24 chin-ups whichever way you get them. What about doing 5, 5, 5, 5 and 4 to get your 24. Perfect also!

Guess what happens when you go past 8, 8 and 8 reps? Say you do 9, 9, and 9 or 10, 10, and 10 or some combination so long as all are above 8 reps. You put your weight belt on and strap a small weight plate to it for extra weight. Doing weighted chin ups will give you a great pump. Not only that, but congratulations are in order. You are now in serious bodybuilding territory.

Training your abs is another exception to the rule of 3 or 4 sets of 8 repetitions. Many of us need many more reps in order to feel any strain.

As part of your experiment, you'll have to find the numbers that suit you best. As some abs exercises are harder than others, you might do 30 crunches on a flat surface and do 15 on an incline surface.

You'll still need to do 3 or 4 different exercises and 3 or 4 sets for each exercise.

The correct number of repetitions is up to you to find out. There's no point in me saying "oh yah just do 25 reps, that'll cover it" when clearly some of you will need to do 50 or more, before you feel pain and push through for a few more.

It's different with the machine exercises, because you can just change the weight. Adjust the weight for a burn at 12 to 15 reps on 'Abb Pulley Crunch' for example.

The other muscle to mention is your calves. Walking around on them your whole life must give them more endurance. You will find that you need a lot more than the standard 8 reps. It will be more like 20 to 30 reps. You still do the 3 or 4 sets per exercise.

MACHINES OR FREE-WEIGHTS

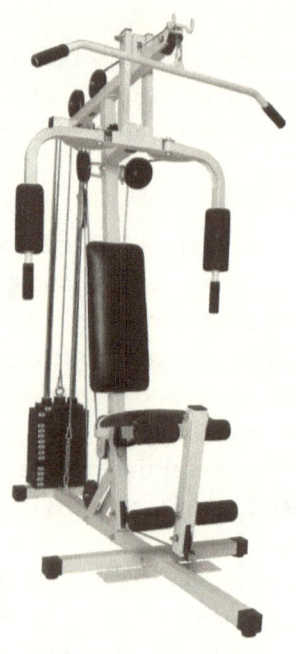

Everyone has seen them advertised on TV. That all in one full body of workout machine. Now don't get me wrong, they are better than nothing, but only when you have no other choice.

Take the bench-press section for example. You lie there and grab the handle's bar, then push. What's wrong with that? A lot. You slide under the handle bars, which won't come down all the way and touch your chest. A restricted motion is the first problem.

You also push up, with the aide of a channel guide. This holds the bar in place so that it can only move up or down. You don't use any muscles to hold it steady. Another restricted motion.

On top of that, many have handle bars with hand grips in one place. You can't hold your hands out wider or bring them in close. Another restricted motion.

When I refer to free-weights, I mean dumbbells and barbells. You are free to move these as you please. When doing free-weights, you must hold them steady, as well as do the pushing or pulling movements.

Holding the free-weights steady adds so much more resistance to the exercises. The added resistance increases your workouts efficiency and in turn your muscle growth.

I know some exercises can only be done using machines. You can't do a complete full body workout without some machine exercises. That's good. But many exercises can be done using either choice. And, my system prefers the free weights over the machines every time. My reason for that is that it's harder doing free-weights.

Take for example the question, what are the three main exercises you can build strength and mass with? I bet every bodybuilder would give exactly the same answer. Which is squats, deadlifts and bench press. And guess what, they are all free-weight exercises.

So for outright strength and size, I will continue to favor a free weight exercise over its machine option.

There are exceptions to my preference for free-weights. I know what you are thinking right now! Why does it have to be so confusing? Or, wish he'd make up his mind. Let me assure you that by the end of the book, everything will fall into place. I'm trying to give you everything I've got.

There are some exceptions like when you have an injury, Say you have a corked thigh muscle.

Squatts are out and probably standing calf raises, plus deadlifts and depending on which leg, lunges are out too.

The machines in a fully stocked gym will allow you to isolate the injured muscles and train around it. Following on with our corked thigh, you can still do standing leg curls, leg extensions and some 1 legged inclined press, plus a toe press for calves. How's that. I'll go into details in a whole chapter on training with an injury.

Another exception I have for machines over free-weights is when you want to isolate a muscle. And why would I want to do that?

To isolate a muscle allows you to directly workout that muscle. By directly, I mean fully fatigue the muscle and get the maximum possible pump for it. We covered that earlier, but your definition is achieved here.

To finish this chapter off, I just want to say that while I prefer free-weights, I can't do a complete workout without both. You get a bigger choice of exercises to do. It allows you to mix it up with a variety which helps keep it interesting.

Not only is it good to shock your muscles with different exercises but it's just also another trick to stop your muscles from getting used to the workout and slowing your growth down.

YOU MUST KNOW THIS

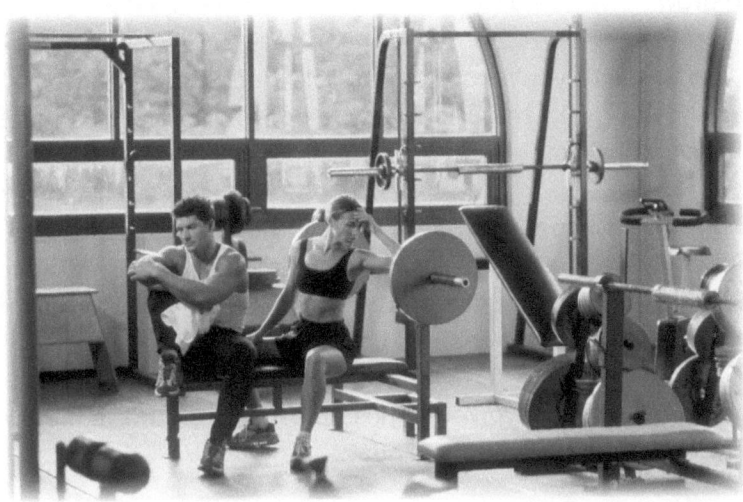

When Do Your Muscles Grow?

If you are going to get the best results from your training, you need to know when your muscles actually grow. When you do your workout, your muscles used become stressed. Your are actually breaking down the muscle tissue.

You are getting a pump, but this isn't muscle growth. Your body needs 48 hours to repair the broken down muscle tissues. The body reacts to the stress by increasing the amount of tissue compared to what existed before you did your workout, and broke down your tissue.

Over several months, you'll notice a definite increase in the size of your muscles. During the many workouts, you have broken down the muscle fibers and they recuperate with a tiny increase in size every time.

So, why do you need to know this? Well, there are two reasons.

Firstly, you must allow your muscles time to grow. The rest period is the ONLY time muscles are able to recover and increase in size.

If you're starting out or super keen for results, it's easy to think you should do the same muscles every day. The fact is, you could actually decrease in size, as your muscles are continually broken down, with no time to grow.

When starting out, you'll cover the whole body between two separate workouts. Half of your muscles could be done for example on Mondays while the other half could be done on Tuesdays.

Following the 48 hours rest rule, you can't do Monday's workout again until Thursday. i.e, break muscles down on Monday, gives 48 hours rest over Tuesday and Wednesday and you're ready to train those muscles again on Thursday. Simple enough, hay.

Likewise with Tuesday's workout. Those muscles rest on Wednesday and Thursday and are ready again on Friday.

Because you're doing two separate workouts, Monday's workout isn't affecting Tuesday's workout and the same with Thursday's and Friday's. 48 hours is the minimum rest you'll need. By the time you get to the advanced game plan, you'll be training so hard that you can only break down (train) each muscle once per week. That's six days for resting and growing.

Secondly, you must know that the weights you lift and push will increase. You can't keep growing with the same weights. Your body will tell you by the fact that you can do the sets and reps easier. If you have to do 10 or 12 to get a burn instead of 8, its time to go up in weight.

None of this can be achieved without proper rest between workouts. The old saying that "less is more" fits perfectly for us bodybuilders.

I KNOW YOU'RE KEEN, BUT DO THIS FIRST!

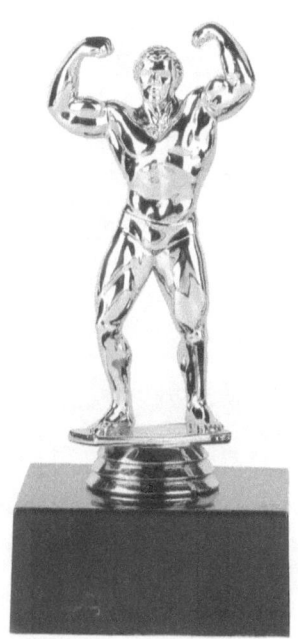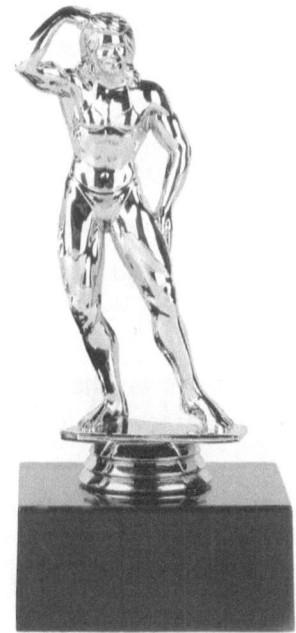

In the long run, this routine is the quickest way for you to get into serious training. I should call it a beginner's routine, but it isn't.

It's the exact routine I've used after any extended periods with no training. And I'll continue to use it following time off my training in the future.

When getting back into training or just starting out, you need to ease it. By spacing the workouts further apart, you're able to cope with sore muscles much better. That is, they won't get sore, so you'll keep turning up to training.

Even splitting the muscles into two separate workouts, A and B requires more than the usual 48 hours rest. This routine gives 72 hours or 3 days rest before the same muscles are used again.

You'll train on one day and rest on the following one. By rotating with two separate workouts gives you the 72 hours of rest for your muscles before that workout is done again.

This is how it looks: **day on / day off routine**

Workouts A and B:

Mon—**A**	Tue	Wed—**B**	Thu	Fri—**A**	Sat	Sun—**B**
Mon	Tue—**A**	Wed	Thu—**B**	Fri	Sat—**A**	Sun
Mon—**B**	Tue	Wed—**A**	Thu	Fri—**B**	Sat	Sun—**A**
Mon	Tue—**B**	Wed	Thu—**A**	Fri	Sat—**B**	Sun

You're going to be given the two separate workouts, A & B, in a later chapter. My point here is to inform you of the game plan.

You can see that over a 4 week period, you'll do 4 workouts the first week, 3 workouts the 2nd week, 4 workouts again in the 3rd week and 3 workouts in the 4th week. Here, the cycle starts over again.

Your sore muscles will appreciate the extra day's rest they get with this game plan. They'll need it because you're going to train hard. You'll be able to train hard and progress quickly to the next level.

You can expect to use this day on / day off routine for 3 months. I would advise against moving onto the second game plan too quickly. Only if you are coming back from an extended rest could you consider 2 months instead of 3.

On the same token, there's absolutely nothing wrong with taking more than 3 months with this routine.

If you are new to bodybuilding, you'll need to lay the foundations as best as you can. The longer you stay on this routine, the better your foundations will be.

What do I mean by foundations? You put a lot of stress on your joints and the associated joining tissues such as cartilage and ligaments. Being patient gives them time to become accustomed to your new routine and the stress you endure. That's why, if you have trained before, your foundations are there and two months is OK.

While I can't be there with you physically, I sure can guide you in this book. The fact there isn't one workout for everyone, including me.

You're getting everything I use. Three different game plans, all up. Call them game plans or workouts, whatever you like.

We have the day on—day off routine, the two day split routine and the single body part routine. Let's keep moving.

GETTING SERIOUS NOW:
THE INTERMEDIATE GAME PLAN

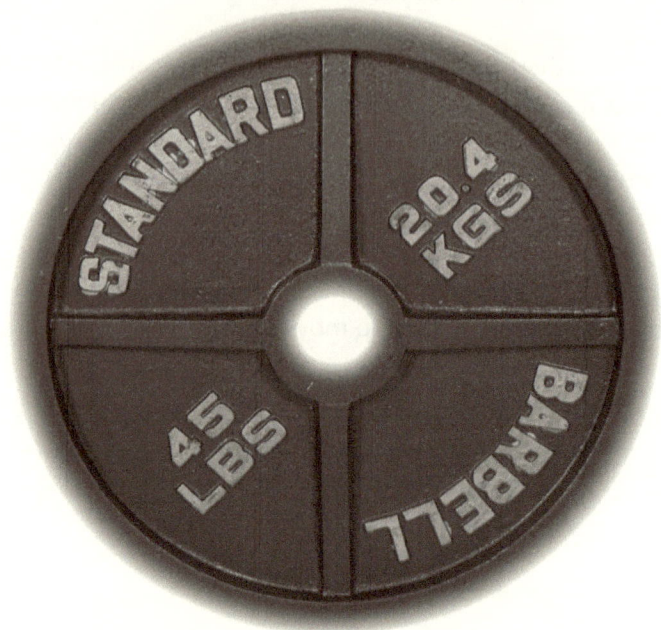

As you might guess, each game plan I give has a higher intensity over the previous one. This 2 day split routine is four days per week.

I have tried all the variations for this routine over the years. From my point of view, there's one variation that's better than the rest. I split the body into eight muscle groups which are legs, chest, triceps, abbs, shoulders, back, biceps and forearms.

Some exercises stimulate muscles in more than one muscle group. To ensure proper rest, it makes sense to keep these muscles in the same workout.

Let me give you some examples; starting with your chest and tricep muscles. When you do bench press, it primarily works your chest, right! But it also works your triceps.

Close-grip bench press is felt in your triceps, but also hits your chest muscles. For this reason, I will always train chest and triceps on the same day and in the same workout.

Another example is back and bicep muscles. As part of my back workout, I love doing various kinds of chin ups. Chin ups work your upper back but it's your biceps that fatigue and cause you to stop. Stress is also placed on your forearms. All these have to be trained on the same day.

Other back exercises like deadlifts, seated pulley rows, lat pull downs, upright rows, and 1 arm rows, all stimulate your biceps, forearm and shoulders.

One last example; Biceps and forearms. When you do barbell or dumbbell curls for your biceps, you'll also get a burn and a pump in your forearms. So these have to be trained together too.

Another heavy influence on my routine is those muscles that I don't want to train together. There are three muscle groups that involve very heavy weights in their routine.

Legs have squatts and incline leg press. Chest has flat bench press. Back has deadlifts. Legs and chest involve pushing movements. The back exercises involve pulling movements.

I want to have enough energy to be able to perform those exercises properly. I can do this if I do the heavy pulling exercises on a separate day to the heavy pushing exercises.

What I'm doing here is giving you the Why. Rather than just saying, do this, do that. I want you to know why I use these variations. Understanding my reasoning will help you stick to it.

After sorting through the muscle groups that I want to train together and the ones that I don't want to, there's only one variation that fits my criteria.

Note: I just want to say that if you train like a pussy, you can use any variations of the muscle groups in your workouts as you like. I didn't get accused of being a pussy; I got accused of being on steroids. If you want similar results with mine, I'm leaving nothing out. All you have to do is read this book and then read it again.

And if you're like me, you might have to read it a 3rd time.

My two day split routine is as follows:

A) Legs, Chest, Chest, Tricep
B) Shoulders, Back, Bicep, Forearm:

Each workout has to be done twice per week. The weekly time table could look like any of these three different combinations, depending on which days you like to train.

Mon—**A**	Tue—**B**	Wed	Thu—**A**	Fri—**B**	Sat	Sun

Or

Mon	Tue—**A**	Web—**B**	Thu	Fri—**A**	Sat—**B**	Sun

Or

Mon	Tue	Wed—**A**	Thu—**B**	Fri	Sat—**A**	Sun—**B**

As with the previous chapter, we're only looking at the game plan. The actual workouts with exercises will be given in a later chapter.

THE ADVANCED GAME PLAN

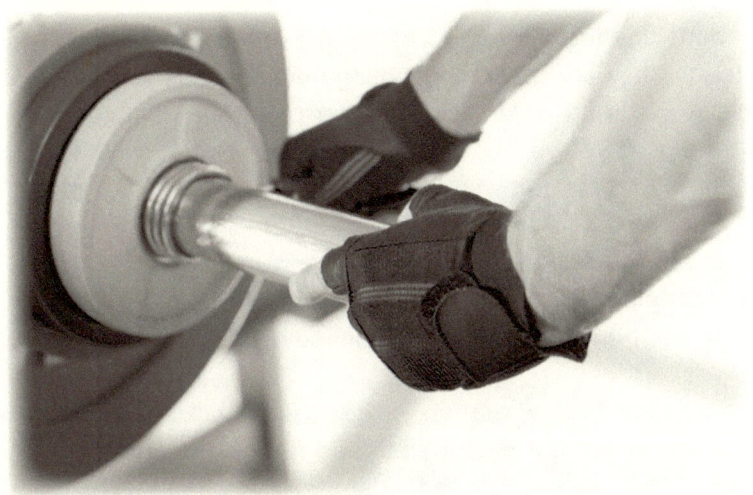

After you have all of my exercises, and my somewhat different approach, the next thing to talk about is how to increase the intensity of your workouts

Here's a list of the things I do for higher intensity, which I will fully explain in this section; Supersets, Exhaust sets, Negative reps, Rest periods and the Five Day Routine.

So far in the book, I've said don't spot ever, ever, ever. I know you must want to know why I don't like spotting or forced reps as some call it. So before we get going on, I'll tell you what my problem is with forced reps.

Some would argue that forced reps or spotting adds intensity to their workout. If everyone else is doing it, then it must be right, seems to suck people in. The fact is, it does add a little intensity, but not enough for my liking.

Using my earlier example where the spotter said "I can't do anymore", it might not be to that extreme all of the time someone spots for their training partner. But it's a fact that while you are spotting your friend, you are losing energy.

That lost energy, wasted on trying to help someone who is fatigued, rep out some more movements, could be put to better use. You get very little out of spotting, but you can lose a whole lot of useful energy.

What about this for a thought. As soon as your spotter grabs the bar or plate etc, they are greatly lightening your load. Its just like dropping your heavy load and picking up a lighter one, then continuing on for a few extra reps. If you've worked up to a certain weight, why let someone lighten it for you? It's not what I do.

If you can push through for one or two or three more reps after you really feel like stopping, you have much more to gain, than reping out a few more with a lighter weight or with someone helping you do it.

To push through in slow motion, or get past a sticking point where the weight stops, or to fight past the burning feeling to get a few extra reps out is going to make spotting redundant.

There is a clear difference and you will come to know of it. Once you feel the difference, you will never let anyone spot you ever again.

The difference is between muscles that are used to being rescued by a spotter. Having the weight intensity lifted as soon as someone grabs it for you, compared to muscles that are used to holding their own; Muscles that are forced to dig deep and deal with that heavy weight on their own.

What this equates to is an incredible leap in your strength and muscle size. I can also report on another benefit. You will feel much safer in the gym, even with heavy weights.

Your safety increases because you get to know what your body can do. Even when you must train on your own, you can still push it hard. Ok, so now let's get back to that list.

SUPERSETS: Pick any two isolation exercises for a muscle. You perform a set of each exercise with no rest between the two sets. It is the lack of rest that increases the intensity.

In your workouts, you will do compound exercises which use heavy weights compared to the isolation exercises. If you try to superset compound exercises, you will risk injury and fatigue from progressive overload.

Take bicep exercises for example. You could start with the compound exercises, heavy dumbbell curl and heavy barbell curl. Finishing off with supersets of restricted curls and pulley curls.

The sets might look like this; 1st superset do 8 reps of restricted curls then immediately follow with 8 reps of pulley curls. Have a short rest and repeat for a total of 3 or 4 sets. It's that simple.

EXHAUST SETS: You do the sets with a second or 2 rests before doing another set, not stopping until you are only able to do 1 or 2 reps.

My favorite exercise for exhaust sets is chin-ups. If I do 9 chin-ups, then 8 chin-ups, then 6 chin-ups, then 5 chin-ups, then 3 chin-ups and 2 chin-ups, that's a total of 33 reps and I'm happy. Just on the last comment I made, my aim is to get down to 2 reps starting at 9, with chin ups and taking a little more rest which is perfectly ok.

Let me explain why I do this. For a normal rep and set count, I want 4 sets of 8 reps, that's a total of 32 reps. Say you can do the following chin-ups 6, 5, 4, 3 , 2 and 2. That is still 22 reps and nothing to sneeze at. I'll even do half reps and stop, then repeat; these half reps are counted as 1. It's just to get the count up.

Another option I use while doing my chin-up exhaust set is to do the different types of chin-ups. They are behind your neck, in front and hands close together with one hand over and one hand under, gripping the bar, or you can grab the bar with both palms facing each other, like holding a tennis racket with 2 hands.

NEGATIVE REPS: These are used when you come to the end of a set and feel like pushing out some more reps. It involves lowering the weight with control and resisting gravity.

To get the weight up, you use cheating methods. Cheating is any means you have to get the weight in the "up" position for you to lower it under control as a negative rep.

Let me give an example, using lying tricep press with a barbell. For this exercise, I like the z-bar, which has like a 'W' bent into the bar instead of just being straight. This bar is just more comfortable on my wrists, so I use it for a lot of my exercises.

For the negative reps, I will just move the bar down to my chest and do a bench press movement just to get it up. Then, bending from the elbows and using my triceps, lower the Z-bar down inline with my forehead. From side on, the whole process moves the bar in a circular motion.

REST PERIODS: You must be aware of how much rest you are taking between sets. If you have a training partner, your rest period is while they are completing their set. The only exception to this is when I'm doing compound exercises.

As compound exercises involve the heaviest weights in your workout, your body might enjoy a little extra rest. The extra rest mostly comes from the time it takes to change the weights around; add plates to the barbell for example.

A gym session can easily fall into a social gathering. Talking in the gym can be your biggest distraction. Apart from a quick 'hello, how are you doing?' I like to avoid too much talking during my training.

Your objective is to get the most out of every workout you do. You just have to look around the gym to know what might seem obvious is overlooked by many people. Get in and get out as quick as you can.

SO WHAT IS WRONG WITH SPOTTING OR FORCED REPS?

Let me start with an example, like most gyms, the one I use has people who are on steroids. From time to time, I have been asked to spot them.

As you know, spotting is not part of my game plan, but each to their own. Any way, I'm standing in front of this guy who's just plain massive. He's doing barbell curls with 90lbs or 40kgs whichever you prefer.

I put, not my whole hand under the bar, but only two fingers each side to help him lift. It was clear to me that this wasn't enough.

When the strain was too much, he had nothing. I was not about to do the curls for him, so he had to stop. I spotted him that way for three sets and he was really struggling. His muscles were not used to such hard work. That guy never asked me to spot him again. So what's my point?

It's like he had no real power. Basically he was all show and no go. I haven't studied exercise physiology, so I can't get all technical for you, but let me give you my point of view.

When I quit spotting and started trying to push the weights on my own, it wasn't long before my muscles became conditioned to it. Where I had to stop before, I could now push through on my own.

The results speak for themselves. Call it an experiment if you like, and based on the results, I drew my own conclusion. And that was, never to spot again.

One time, I was doing seated dumbbell press for my shoulders and sitting next to me was the guy I spotted in the above example.

By that time, I'd worked up to 100lbs dumbbell shoulder press. The guys next to me were using 70lbs dumbbells and even at that weight they were spotting each other.

I caught wind of someone complaining and heard one of them say "don't worry about what they're doing, just concentrate on what you're doing" That was kind of cool.

A final word on why I hate spotting. You are missing out on the massive difference in strength and growth.

How can you possibly get deep tissue growth and true power if you are rescued every time it gets a little hard? You can't and you won't, so don't. All your spotters out there need to harden up! No I'm kidding. But you won't break through those barriers until you stop doing it (spotting).

A WORD ON FORM

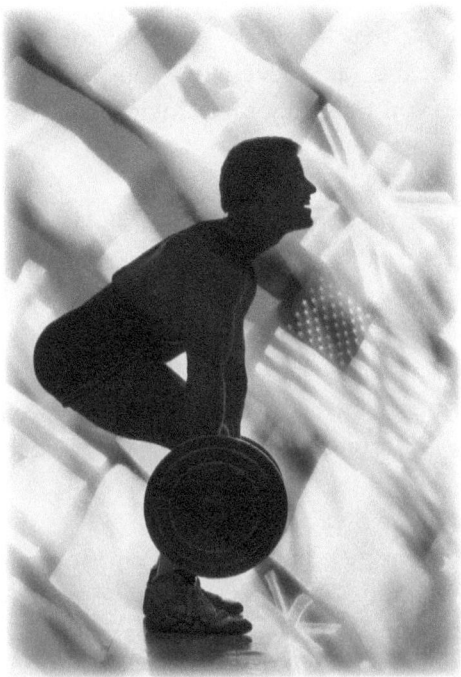

We've reached the final chapter, before we start putting it all together, form or technique as some of you call it, is the last thing I need to address. If you are conscious of doing your movements with the correct form, you'll get so much more out of your training.

The reason you get more out of your workouts is that it's harder to train with correct form. I see a lot of people taking shortcuts and basically cheating.

Whether from impatience for results or some other reasons, I've seen people trying to use weights that are way too heavy. By doing that, you need to swing the barbell or dumbbell, to get it up.

Also, lowering the weight too quickly and not resisting gravity is also cheating. You want to have full control up and down with no swinging.

Just to clarify swinging for you, it means you might rock your body and arms or even your legs in the same direction as you want to move the weight. Cheating this way makes it much easier to do your reps.

If you cheat with your form, you'll reduce your gains. Say you have a training partner at the same level with you. That is, you both use the same weights when you train together. One of you uses correct form and the other mostly cheats.

The one who cheats will very quickly fall behind in the weights being used and in appearance. Who ever does correct form will develop rippling muscle and get stronger quickly.

In an earlier chapter, I talked about the experiment. This chapter gives the emphasis you might need to understand why you need to do the experiment. It's so important to take time to find your 8 rep weight for every exercise.

You won't walk into the gym and start training to your maximum using the correct form without first doing the experiment. Which, to quickly repeat, means finding the exact weight for each exercise that allows you to just get 8 reps out.

If you can do only 6, it's too heavy and doing 10 means it's too light. When you start off, doing three sets might turn out something like this; 8 reps, then 7 reps, then 7 or even 6 reps on the 3rd set. That's all good. After several weeks, you'll get to three sets of 9 reps (9, 9, 9) and it is then time to increase the weight. (10, 10, 10) is ok too.

As short as this chapter is, it is one of the most important chapters in this book. It's going to make a massive difference in your results if you keep "correct form" in the back of your mind while training.

Now we're moving into the exercises. I'm giving you a description of more than 50 exercises that I use. I've broken the body parts into 8 chapters, covering exactly 54 exercises.

LEG EXERCISES

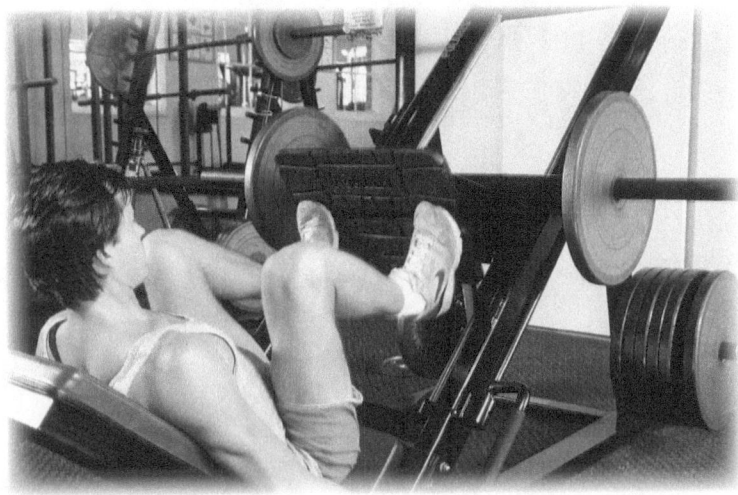

These are the legs exercises I use. You'll do all of them when training your legs.

SQUAT: I never do squats without a weight-belt. In a standing position, and facing the squat rack, duck under the barbell so it rests across the back of your lower neck. When you have the weight in control, take several half steps back, just to clear the rack.

The bar needs to be low enough so that when you straighten your legs, it lifts the bar off the squat rack. You also want your feet facing straight ahead and about shoulder width apart.

You must keep your back straight the whole time. A trick for this is to just look at a spot about 2 feet above your head, on the wall in front of you. If the rack is in an open space, just focus on any high spot during the movement.

When squatting down, don't go too far. When your thighs are almost parallel to the ground, that's low enough. That's it!

INCLINE LEG PRESS: This exercise can only be done on the special machine designed specifically for this exercise.

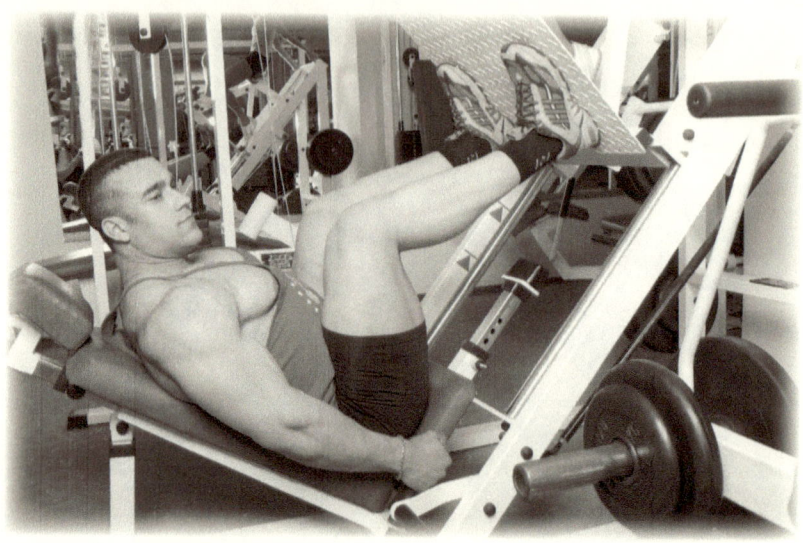

In a seated position, you use your legs to push the press machine which moves on a gentle slope of about 25 degrees. At the start of your first rep, you take the strain and move the safety pins outwards with your hands. When you have finished your set, you roll the pins inwards; this holds the weight.

You want your feet apart on the push plate. Very similar to how you place your feet for a squat. Only lower the press machine until your thighs nearly touch your abs. Any lower and you're straining your knees. There's no more to it.

TOE PRESS: This exercise is done on the leg press machine, the same one you use for incline leg press.

It's a calf muscle exercise and easily done after the above exercise. Sitting in the machine, you take the weights with your legs and release the safety pins. Then, straighten your legs and lock your knees stiff.

Using only the pads of your feet, just below your toes, push the plate. The movement is only done by rolling your ankle joint, your hips and knees don't move; there's no other leg movement. At full extension, it's like you're on your tippy toes. Another way to look at it is like you're using an accelerator with both feet.

As with the leg press, when you're finished, roll the safety pins into place and climb out, or rest until your next set. If you're on your own, it's easier to just stay in position. That's it.

LEG EXTENSION: This exercise is also done on a specially designed machine. First, you set the weight you want by inserting the pin. Then you may have to adjust the pad which rests against your shins. Have it rest in the middle of your shin. Then take a seat with your shins resting behind the pads and your hands holding the handgrips beside your seat.

The movement requires that your top be extended from your knees. Using both legs together, you raise your lower legs towards the horizontal position. This raises the weights on the pulley behind you.

The exercise works your quads which are basically your thigh muscles in your upper legs. It will give your legs definition. We don't want to turn you into a stork, with big upper body and pencil legs.

LEG CURLS: This exercise is done on another specially designed machine. You can only do one exercise with this machine, and that's leg curls.

It works your hamstrings or the back of your upper legs. Again, you first have to set the weight you want with the pin. Standing up, you'll hold the T-bar in front for support.

You do one leg at a time. The leg that you want to work will have its calf muscle resting on the pad. You raise your foot behind you, performing the leg curling movement. You will need to do the movement with control. By that I mean, slowly up and slowly down, not letting the weight down too quick.

For all of the pulley exercises, for legs or any muscle group, always raise and lower with full control. Don't let the weight slam back down, keep the strain and have control of the whole movement up and down.

STIFF LEG DEADLIFT: For this exercise, you only need a barbell with a fairly light weight. What's light? Only use 1/4 to 1/3 of your body weight, but no more.

You do this while standing up, and as I said, you must have your legs stiff, no bending at all, once you've picked up the bar.

Hold the bar about the shoulder width apart while standing with your feet close together. It's very important to keep your back straight during the exercise. That's easily done if you just look up during the exercise. Just pick a high spot and focus on it during your set. The spot can be anything above your head, near the roof, high on a wall; whatever.

If you did look down, it tends to arch your back. This is when it's possible to pull a muscle. So just keep your back straight by looking up during the whole movement and you'll be fine; no injuries ever.

While it's mostly stretching your hamstrings, you will work your lower back muscles at the same time.

STANDING CALF RAISES: Here's another exercise with a special machine made just for it. As the name suggest, it's for your calf muscles.

Before you start, set the weight you want with the pin. Stand on the small platform with just your toes and pads of your feet on the platform.

Duck down and rise up so the pads are resting on your shoulders and hold the hand grips for balance.

During the exercise, you should keep your knees locked stiff and only bend from your ankles. Rise up like you're on tippy-toes and lower down and repeat. By hanging your heels over the edge, it gives you a greater range of motion to work the muscle more effectively.

That's it; it's really that simple. I know some of these hardly need explaining, but if you haven't used gym machines before, you'll be glad I included these paragraphs.

SITTING CALF RAISES: Here's another calf muscle exercise and another machine that's made just for it.

When you sit on the seat with your feet on a similar platform to the standing calf machine, you can move the padded t-bar over your knees.

If it's sitting too high above your knees or it's too low to move into position above your knees, there's a pin that allows you to adjust the height, so just set it to your liking. Once that's done, you're ready to add some weights.

As part of this little machine, there's a stand that holds it up when you have finished your reps. The stand is connected to a little handle on one side of your seat. You just have to hold the stand up out of the way during your set. As soon as you see the machine, you'll see exactly what I mean. No more to it.

CHEST EXERCISES

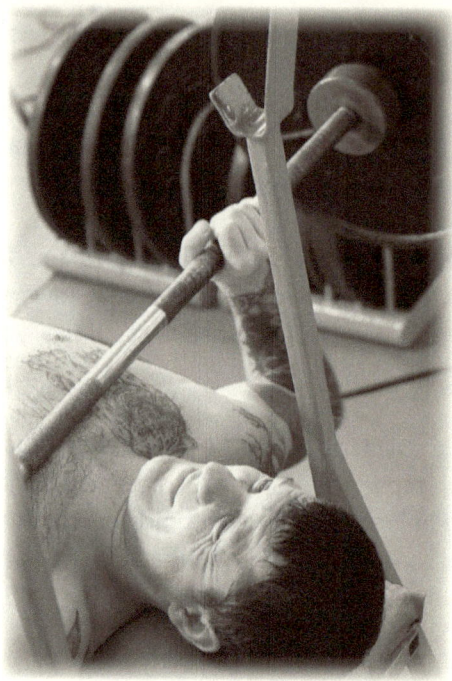

BENCH PRESS: There's not much to say about this one. It's most peoples' favorite exercise, me included.

Be sure to position your chest and shoulders directly under the bar, so you're doing a straight lift, up and down. If you didn't position yourself under the bar, you are lifting on an angle and losing power through bad technique.

The other thing is, don't bounce the bar off your chest but keep control of the movement the whole time. The bars are usually marked with a place to grab it, so if anything, you can grab the inside of the grip. They are usually two hands width long, so just hold closer than out wide.

PECK DECK: Done on a special peck-deck machine. It is one of the easiest to use in the whole gym.

First, just select your weight by inserting the pin in the hole for the weight you want. You also have an option to adjust the seat height.

You'll push against the pads with your forearms; in a bent position. The pads are about a foot long, so they rest on your arm from your elbow to your wrist.

I find it much better to do both arms at the same time. You can also try a brief pause and hold the weight for a second or two. It can give you a better pump, but you won't need to do that on every rep in your set.

BENCH FLY: You do this exercise lying on a flat bench with a light dumbbell in each hand.

It's important to have your arms only slightly bent at your elbows and to keep them in that position for the whole set.

When your arms are out to your side, have your palms facing up to the roof. But when you raise them up together, roll your wrists outward on every rep. So at the top of the movement, you're looking at your palms.

This technique gives you a better squeeze or pump for your chest muscles. And because you're only using light dumbbells, you can do the squeeze every rep with no problem.

INCLINE PRESS: You have some options with this exercise. You can use a barbell with an incline bench with arms that hold the bar between sets. Or, I prefer to use an adjustable bench without the attachment arms, and to use dumbbells instead of a bar. I like the bench set at about 30' (degrees).

I need to tell you how I get ready, using dumbbells. You don't need your training partner to help you do this.

Stand at the end of your bench so that when you're ready, you can sit and lean back easily.

When you pick the dumbbells up, rest one end on each thigh so as they stand tall after you sit down. You can lift them up, one at a time, using your knee to give the dumbbell a little push, by raising your knee to jack it up. It works wonders for heavy dumbbells.

Once you have both dumbbells up at your shoulders, lay back, and you're ready to start. Always push both dumbbells at the same time.

If you have worked your way up to heavy dumbbells, you can unload using the same technique with your knees.

To unload, bring a knee up, and rest the dumbbell on your thigh. When your foot is back on the ground, the dumbbell will be standing tall on one end. Do the same with both dumbbells.

If you're putting the dumbbells on the floor, be sure to keep looking high as you lower them to the floor. Arch your back holding heavy dumbbells and you could pull a muscle. Always bend from your knees and never lean over; always keep your torso upright. Use your legs and when in doubt, guess what? Yep, use your legs.

I just want to give some more safety measures. You can pick the heaviest dumbbells off the floor that you're going to train on with no problem, provided you do it right. Do it by squatting down over the dumbbells and grabbing them with your back straight. All the lifting is done with your legs. So, lowering the weights all the way to the ground is done exactly the same way. Squat by bending your legs with your back straight. Sorry to go on about it, but I've seen some pretty bad techniques in the gym.

DUMBELL PRESS: You're going to need a flat bench for this one. It's just like barbell bench press, but using dumbbells.

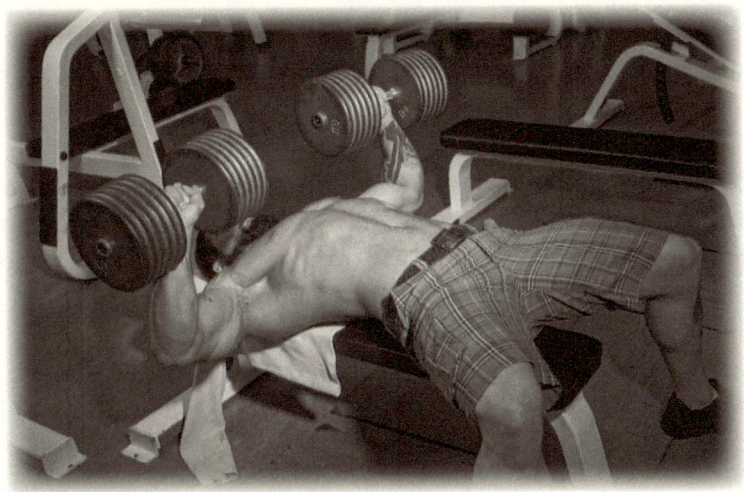

You need a training partner to load you up for this exercise. It's too far to role back with two heavy dumbbells. Your training partner will load you up once you're lying down and ready to receive the dumbbells one at a time.

You do the same movement as you would with the barbell. No twisting of your wrists etc, just straight up and down presses.

When you're finished, you'll need your partner to unload you, by taking the dumbbells one at a time.

CABLE CROSSOVERS: You do this one while standing in the middle of the cable crossover machine.

Go over to one side, grab the pulley cable handle, then walk over to the other side, still holding the first handle, and grab the second handle. Move back to the middle, so you have equal tension from both cables.

You'll start with your arms out to your side at shoulder height. Bring both arms in at the same time. Your arms remain slightly bent. Push each hand across your body so that your arms cross over each other.

Your hands will be down around your abs region when you have fully crossed your hands over.

Pause for a moment at the cross over position before letting the cables pull your arms back to the starting position. The pause is a quick flex of your chest muscles.

I use all seven of these chest exercises, but never on the same day. Three or four exercises for any one workout. With the variety you can get by changing the exercises around, you can keep shocking your muscles. Never let your muscles get used to your routine and become stale.

Constantly, push your muscles and they will grow at light speed. That goes for all of the muscle groups. Mix up the routine with the different exercises I give you.

You might even have some of your own that you want to include, that's fine. It also stops boredom. A little variety keeps it interesting for you too.

TRICEP EXERCISES

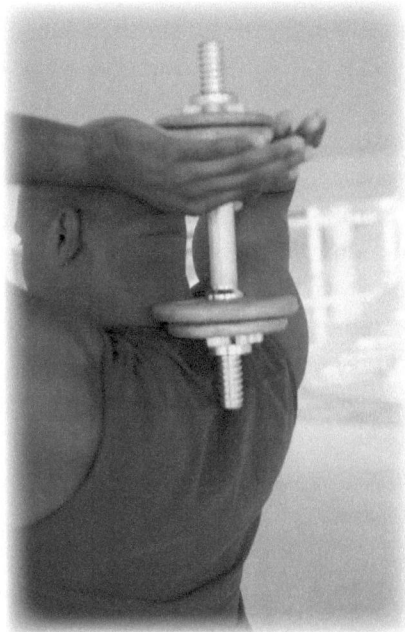

Z-BAR PRESS: This is my favorite because it always gives me the best pump. That's because Z-Bar press hits your triceps just right. It's similar to bench press but still unique enough.

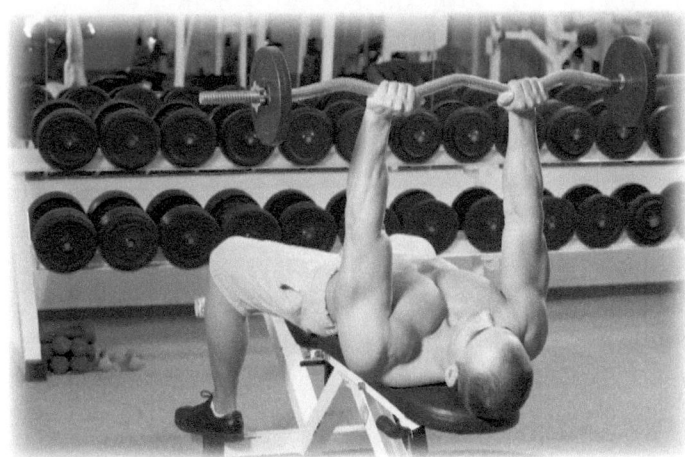

You need the same bench as bench press and you do it while lying down. The rest is different. You don't use a straight barbell, but use the short bent bar. Some call it and E-Z bar.

They're more comfortable on your wrists than the straight bar. You hold the bar with your hands 6 to 8 inches apart. Nice and close.

Lying on your back, take the bar out of the rack and take the weight (hold it steady). For this exercise, you only bend from your elbows. Lowering the bar towards your forehead and keeping your upper arms stiff and still pointing upwards. Remember, only bend from your elbows, using your triceps to raise and lower the bar.

If you go too heavy, it's very hard to keep your upper arms stiff, and as you lower the bar, your elbows will tend to move out to the side.

You'll get more out of it if you keep strict form, so lower your weight and keep your elbows in—always!

Sometimes, you'll want to fully fatigue your triceps with this exercise. If you're using a weight that you can do 8 reps with, there is a way to get a few more reps, to really blast your triceps, with this exercise. Here's how you do it.

After the 8 reps, your muscles should be totally spent, but there's still something you can do. Lower the bar in the normal way, using the last bit of energy in your triceps. Then to get the bar up again, lower your elbows and do a bench press movement. You can easily push it up again.

Lower it down with the stiff upper arms over your forehead, and push it back up as a bench press movement. So you're doing half the Z-Bar press to totally tax the last energy your triceps have.

The lowering part is normal Z-bar movement and raising part is a bench press movement. Repeat the movement for 3, 4 or 5 more reps after your last set.

I would normally do this; two sets of 8 reps normally, then with the last two sets, use the half bench press / half Z-bar press reps for as many extra as you can, after the 8 normal reps. If I did 3 extra reps, I'm looking at a total of 11 reps for that set. Sometimes you might only do 1 extra. There's no set rule here, any extra is the right answer.

LAT MACHINE PULLDOWN: I do this exercise on most triceps days also. It's great for isolating my triceps. By that, I mean working just that muscle and getting a good pump from the exercise.

So what is it? It's another machine exercise that you'll find in all fully equipped gyms. You do it while standing; with your two hands holding a small bar in a close grip. While pushing down, you must lock your elbows so that only your forearms are moving. The only joints that move are your elbows.

In a controlled motion, you push down and keep control as you let your arms raise again. I find it beneficial to use different bars for this exercise.

One of the hardest to use is a short bar with a spinning handle. By harder I mean more beneficial. By beneficial, I mean taking the shortest possible path to success.

KICKBACKS: This is a dumbbell exercise. You'll stand and bend over with your torso parallel to the ground. Holding one dumbbell, you can easily support yourself with the other hand by holding a chair or bench.

The only movement is from your elbow. The upper arm is held stiff, by your side, making it parallel to the ground also.

Holding the dumbbell, you'll bend and straighten your arm. As you bend your arm, it's pointing to the ground. You then straighten it until it's parallel to the ground.

The hardest part is to straighten your arm while holding the dumbbell. You're pushing against gravity here. This is an advanced exercise that will really give your triceps a hard workout.

DUMBELL DIPS: As it sound, it's another dumbbell exercise. You do it while sitting down.

You must pick up the dumbbell with both hands. There's a little knack to it, let me explain how.

First, you're not trying to fit both hands on the little bar between the plates. Here's how you grab it.

Your first step is to lock your thumbs together. Have a practice! Then, whichever thumb is on top, the fingers of that hand will also be on top of the fingers of the other hand.

By locking your thumbs, when you place your fingers from one hand on top of the other, what do you notice? I'll tell you. Your fingers sit at 90 degrees from one hand to the other

It forms a cuff for both palms to hold a plate on any one side of the dumbbell. The dumbbell handle passes through the hole formed between your two hands held together.

When you're holding the dumbbell with both hands this way, it is standing upright throughout the whole set.

I actually stand the dumbbell up on one end, just before I pick it up. Holding it with one hand, then just slide the other hand in, laying the top hand across the top of the other hand at 90 degrees. Lock your thumbs together and you're ready to lift it into position.

OK, now you can grab it, what do you do with it? Glad you asked. Bending from your elbows, you raise it right above your head and lower it down behind your head.

You can use a moderate weight for this, so don't be shy. Try different weights until you get the right weight. By that, I'm talking about chapter 4 and how you must experiment with your weights to get the most out of your workout.

PARALLEL BAR DIPS: Most gyms have these bars and they are usually attached to a chin up bar. The dip bar is a great exercise for your chest and triceps.

All you need to do is stand between the two horizontal bars and step up or push yourself to the starting position.

That being the case, with both arms straight by your side, hold your weight off the ground. To do the exercise, just lower yourself down and push up again.

A few points need to be made here. When you're starting out, you will not need to lower yourself far, for the exercise to work.

After some weeks, you'll be lowering yourself right down to the bars before pushing back up to the straight arm position.

There are two variations for this exercise. If you sit your chin on your chest throughout the movement, it focuses the strain on your chest. And if you lift your head and chin up, looking towards the ceiling, it focuses the strain on your triceps. I usually do a few sets of each variation.

1-ARM TRICEP PRESS: Here's another great exercise that you'll get definition from. You need to experiment with the weight so that you can just do 8 to 10 reps and its burning like fire, on the last few reps.

In a seated position, grab one dumbbell. As a guide, it's about 1/3 of the weight you use for dumbbell bicep curls. Raise your dumbbell straight up, above your head, with arms straight and stretching to the sky.

Bending from your elbow, lower the dumbbell down behind your head. Only your lower arm (elbow to hand) moves and your upper arm (elbow to shoulder) stays pointing skyward.

As your weights get heavier, you'll find it more comfortable to clasp or hold the exercising triceps with the other hand. Here's how I get started. One arm grabs the dumbbell and the other hand forms a cuff and clasps over your triceps. i.e, your thumb doesn't wrap around your arm; it's part of the cuff that supports your triceps.

With the hands in position, raise your arms above your head and begin. The dumbbell is not lowered behind but across your body, passing behind your head; as easy as that.

ABDOMINAL EXERCISES

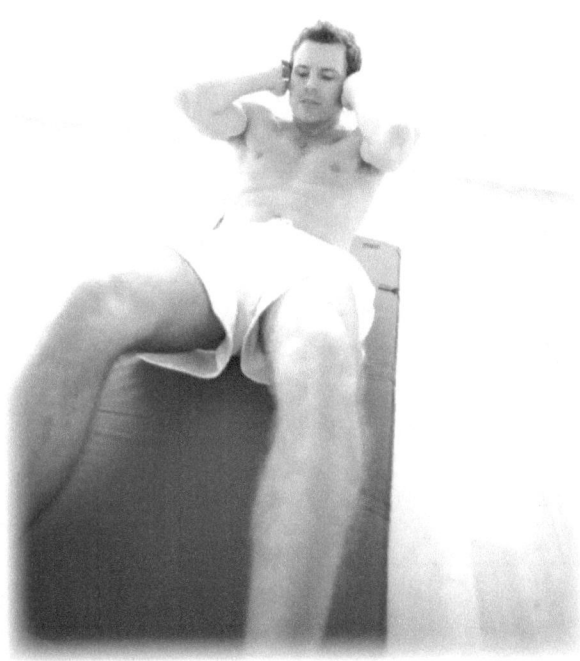

CRUNCHES: Lie on your back with the knees bent. You really need to lift only your shoulders off the ground. I rest my hands on my thighs and slide my hands up as I crunch. It's not a big range of movement.

You can do variations of crunches by putting your legs in different positions i.e knees bent, legs straight, both legs up in the air or one leg up and the other down. Crunches are easily done and no equipment is required.

INCLINE SITUPS / CRUNCHES: You need an incline bench with foot straps for this exercise. It's hard because the incline exaggerates your body weight when you're raising your torso. No more to it.

LEG RAISES: You can hold onto the chin up bar or use the dip bars for this exercise. All you're doing is raising your legs up to some point past a parallel position while holding, for a moment, at the top of the movement.

Both legs are straight and moved together, only bending from your hips. That's it.

KNEE UPS: You can do these lying on a bench or like you're doing leg raises. All you're doing is raising your knees towards your chest. Raise both knees at the same time. This is a lower impact version of the Leg raises exercise.

PULLEY CRUNCH: Any pulley machine that you can pull from high up, towards the ground is what you need. I usually use the rope handles attached to the pulley cable.

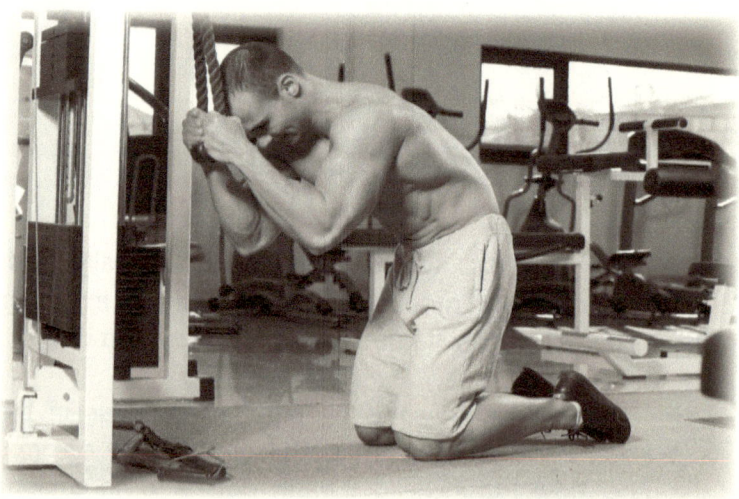

Position yourself on your knees in front of the pulley machine. Hold the rope handles with each hand resting on your chest and the rope running past each ear. As you crunch forward, you're pulling on the weights.

SITUP CHAIR: These new devices give me the best ab workout I can get. What I like is how I can adjust the impact by moving the pin to a different setting.

Sitting on a chair with back support and crunching from a position level to the floor is effective. But when you lower the position past the ground level, it increases the intensity much more.

By increasing the range of movement and stretching of your abbs gives you a great workout. You never do all of these in one workout; 3 or 4 are enough and you should swap them as you like.

SHOULDER EXERCISES

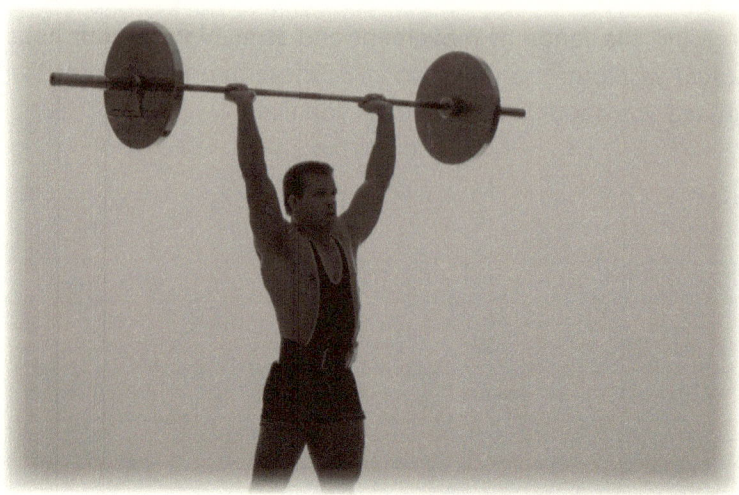

BEHIND NECK PRESS: There's a special piece of equipment for this. A padded seat with a rack to hold the barbell and some have a platform for your safety guy to stand on. I can't call him / her my spotter because I don't ever use them, so its safety guy or girl, ok.

What a power house exercise, one of my favorites. You'll get massive shoulders doing this exercise, I promise you that. Even when you're stuck half way, your safety guy/girl must show restraint and let you slowly push it up.

Then try for another rep. You might get it or you might not. You must keep going until your safety guy has to help you place the bar back on the rack. Pushing yourself this way will make you very strong and get you massive quickly.

A quick note on pushing yourself this way: Every time you muster the courage to push past the sticking points, that one extra rep is worth a whole week of normal training, even longer.

After a while, your muscles will have more deep power to be able to do this. I call these reps the "Slow Motion" reps, as you will see; it's as if they are done in slow motion.

To some one watching, it looks like you're stuck, but after a pause, you will slowly move the weight. Someone nearby, who's used to spotting, will try to jump in and grab the weight. Many times I have had to say "leave it" to an eager beaver thinking they are helping me out. No thanks, NO SPOTTING.

This is so much different to the old Spotting method that most people use. Someone used to spotting takes a while to be able to adjust to this new approach. Spotting gives you shallow muscle depth.

When your muscles are fatigued they have nothing, zero, zilch, nadda left for another rep. But, train without spotting, forcing yourself to take the full weight the whole time, which gives you deep tissue strength allowing you to just power through, often in slow motion, but you still have this power you would never have experienced before, while training with spotting.

DUMBELL PRESS: I like to sit on a padded chair with complete back support. You'll use heavy dumbbells for this exercise.

With palms facing forward, push both dumbbells above your head at the same time.

When you lower your dumbbells, you may feel more comfortable to role your wrists in, so your palms are facing your head after you've lowered them to the top of your shoulders.

Then, when you're ready to push up, as you do, your wrists will pivot and at the top of the movement, with hands straight above your head, your palms are facing forward again.

Often the last few reps will be in the classic slow motion, as I force them up to complete the set.

My problem with spotting is that Mr. Spotter wants to jump in before you even exert yourself. And, by grabbing the weight, they are greatly reducing the load. Spotters will never be able to push through sticking points; their muscles are conditioned to be rescued by their training partners.

There is no need for the deep tissue to develop, because it's never used.

There's no satisfaction like being able to push through a sticking point when you're being watched and it appears you're trying to lift too much. I've had people sitting near me say to each other "what's this guy doing" then move away when they watch me push through the sticking point. This happens when some guys are puffed up on roids, looking bigger than me, and when I use heavier weights than they can, with no spotting, they don't like it.

How many times have I heard, "you worry about what you're doing, don't worry about what he's doing". He, being me. This happens when I'm next to some guys doing the same exercise, they are bigger than me, but I'm using heavier weights. Steroid freaks can be bitchy sometimes, hay.

I'm pouring my heart into this book. You know I'm telling the truth. Where would I get the insights to make it all up? I've lived it, that's where it comes from. I feel like I'm entitled to write this book.

It's for people like you who will take it and use it and find out for yourself. I hope you provide some feedback on your success and experiences.

UPRIGHT ROW: You'll do this exercise with a barbell and be standing up. You need to grab the barbell with your hands close together, say 6 to 8 inches apart.

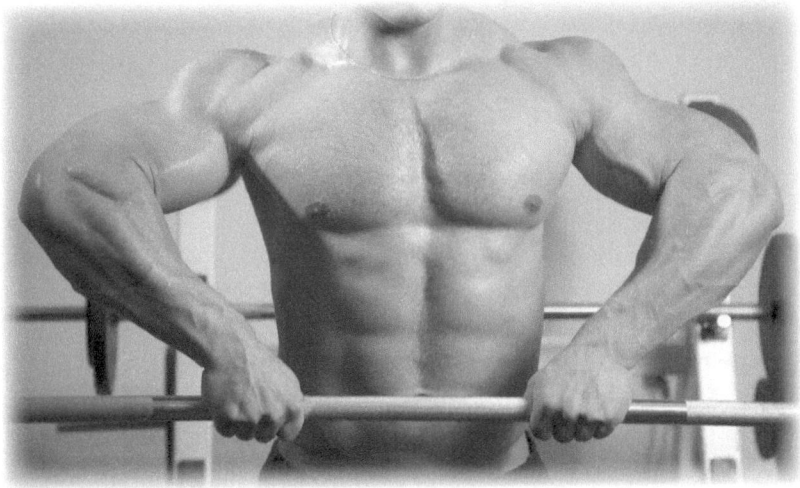

Which way do you grab it, you ask? Grab it with your palms facing down. If that's a little confusing, let me elaborate. If you're doing barbell curls, you're grabbing the bar underneath, which means your palms are facing upward. The opposite way is to grab the bar from the top, with the palms facing down. See the difference? Good.

Right, you've grabbed the bar, palms facing down. Now, lift it up, to just under your chin and let it down again. That's one rep.

I find it better to slightly bend my knees. It keeps me from rocking during the set. Rocking can give you leverage and help; you cheat. Cheat at Poker, not in your bodybuilding.

One last point is to do the reps with control, which means not too fast and not too slow. Don't just let gravity pull the bar down, but lower it with control.

BENT SIDE LATERALS: This is a dumbbell exercise done while standing but bent over. Start with both arms hanging down towards the floor. With arms slightly bent through the whole movement, raise the dumbbells out to your side. Both arms are moved at the same time. Keep control of the speed for the whole rep, just like you do for upright rows.

SIDE LATERALS: This is a variation to Bent Side Laterals except that it's done while standing up. Start with your hands holding the dumbbells down by your waist or even touching in front of your lower abs.

Raise both arms together until they are just past your shoulder height, pausing for a second, before lowering down slowly. Between these two side lateral exercises, bent side laterals and side laterals, you're hitting all three deltoid muscles in your shoulders. That's front, side and rear deltoids.

They're done with light weights but are good for sculpting your muscles, giving you good definition in your shoulders.

BACK AND TRAP EXERCISES

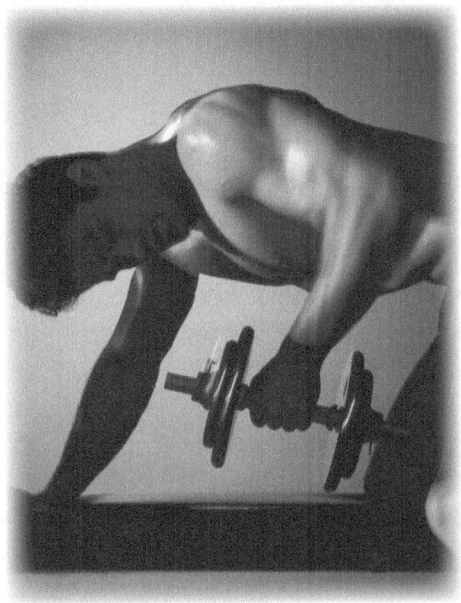

DEAD-LIFT: This exercise will greatly improve your strength and size, making it one of my favorites. It is done with a barbell and while standing up.

Grab the bar at shoulder width apart, with one hand over the grip and one hand under the grip. That's right, you use opposite grips on this exercise.

The bar will be picked off the floor, with feet at shoulder width apart and toes pointing straight ahead. You must keep your back upright when picking up the bar. Do this by only bending at your knees.

As you lift, it helps keep your back upright if you look at some point above your head and keep your head up while looking at that point throughout the whole set. This exercise uses heavy weights, so you must never arch your back or lean forward.

I'm putting so much into the techniques to give you years of injury free training.

Never, ever do this exercise without a weight-belt. Some people also think you need to do this exercise on a platform or box.

No way, don't do it, the extra range only hurts your knees. There's plenty or range of movements lifting the bar while standing on the floor.

Just push up with your legs until they (your legs) are straight. Your arms will be straight also. It's too much weight to try bending your arms. Keeping your chin up and eye's focused on a high point, lower the bar back down, touching the ground is fine, then repeat.

If you're doing 4 sets, do 2 sets with your grip in one position then change for the last 2 sets i.e, left hand over grip / right hand under grip for 2 sets, and then swap grips around.

LAT-PULLDOWN: This is a seated exercise, done with one of the pulley machines. There are a variety of bars to try, so use whatever feels best for you. Set the pin at your starting weight, lock your knees under the pad and you're ready to start pulling the bar down, behind your head.

When you've pulled it down as far as you can behind your head, hold for a second or two, before letting it up again. Easy stuff.

PULLEY ROW: Here's another pulley machine exercise, done in a kind of rowing position. You need a short bar for this exercise.

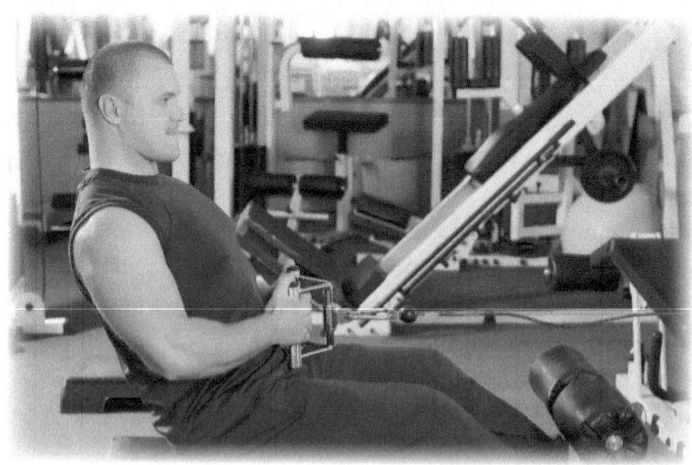

At all times, your back must be straight, never arching forward, or rounding your shoulders. Your upper body (torso) might rock a little, but never let the weight pull you right forward.

Your arms pull the weight. Pull the bar into your sternum or upper abs region. When you've pulled it all the way in, flex your lats which are your upper back under your arm-pits. Pause and flex for a second or two. And never forget to wear your weight belt. That's all there is too it.

CHIN-UPS: These are hard and nobody seems to like them. I love them and you also will.

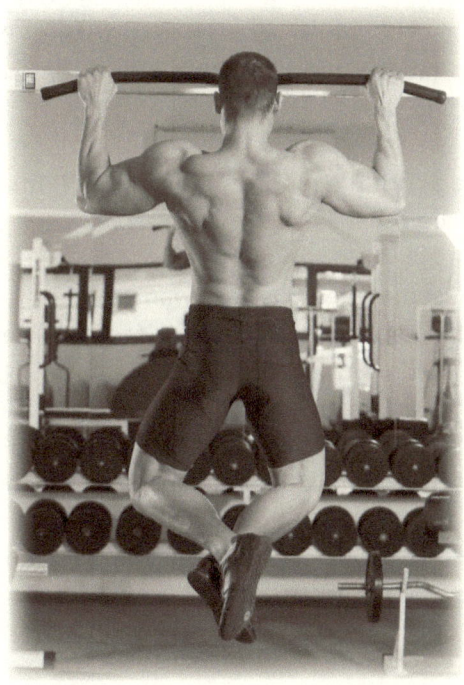

You should grab the bar with your palms facing away from you. If you grab it with palms facing inwards, it's more like a bicep curl.

Don't do bicep chin ups, do back exercise chin ups. Your lats love these.

When you start, you might get 3, 4 or 5 reps out. Even 2 reps are ok. It just means that if you really want 3 sets of 8 reps for a total of 24, you'll be doing more than 3 sets. If you're doing 2, 3, 4 or 5 reps instead of 8, ok. Say you can do 4 reps each set and then then you need 6 sets of 4; to get to the magic number 24, whatever your rep count is, just divide it by 24 to get the number of sets you need.

When I'm fully done and can't go anymore, I still do a few more single rep sets or even half rep sets. That's right, do half a chin up and stop for a short recovery and repeat 2 or 3 or 4 times. Half reps still count as 1.

Also, 24 is the minimum, so after a while, you'll be doing a pyramid count, such as 8, 7, 6, 5, 4, 3, 2, and several 1's for a total of 36 to 40 reps. The point is to train to fatigue and know that 1 or 2 reps sets are very good for your bodybuilding.

I'll be talking more about the range of reps in the "Putting It All Together" chapter. But there are other exercises; you can do a 1, 2 or 3 rep set.

Take bench press; sometimes you just want to see how much you can push out for 1 or 2 reps. It is a powerful feeling. The same goes with deadlifts.

BENT ROW: This exercise is done with a barbell and performed while standing and bent over from your waist, knees slightly bent.

Holding the barbell at shoulder width apart and starting with your arms hanging down, you pull the bar towards your ab region. The bar is held with palms facing down, i.e, in an overhand grip.

At all times, you must wear your weight belt. Don't bend over the ground level. Bend over just past 45 degree's is good. Having bent knees takes the strain off your back.

SHRUGS: This is done in a standing position, while holding heavy dumbbells. Your arms are by your side and kept straight; never bend them.

Lift your shoulders up, trying to touch your ears with your shoulders. Pause for a second at the top of the movement. Lower your shoulders back down, and that's one rep.

1-ARM ROW: I like to do this exercise on a padded bench. It's done with a dumbbell and uses one arm at a time.

You need one knee on the bench and the same side arm also on the bench, holding you up. That arm is out straight while leaning on the bench. Your other foot is on the floor, with your leg holding most of the balance. You're half on the bench, half off it.

Your spare arm is holding the dumbbell. Holding the dumbbell with your arm stretched towards the floor, you're ready to start. Pull the dumbbell up towards your lower chest. Try to flex your lats at the top of the movement. And don't forget your weight belt.

BICEP EXERCISES

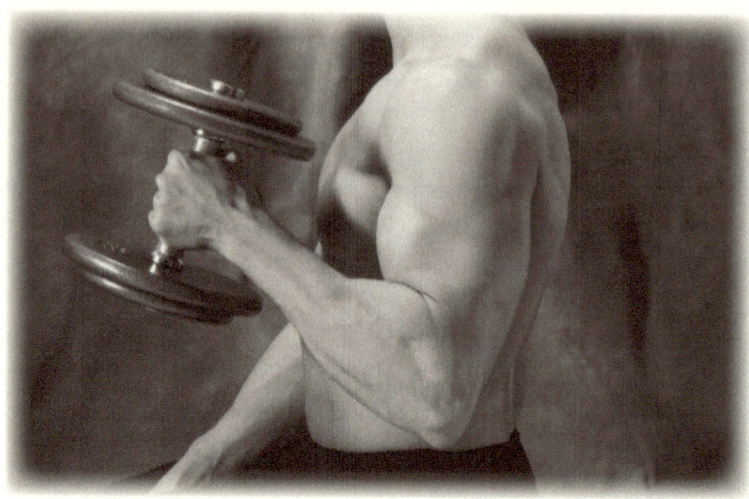

DUMBELL CURL: As the dumbbells sit on the floor, they are flat to the ground. During your dumbbell curls, keep them at a flat level with the ground.

I prefer to do my dumbbell curls while sitting on a padded seat. Do not swing them up. People going too heavy usually need to do this. Controlled, move up and down, and push through the burn for one or two reps.

BARBELL CURL: I like to do this exercise while standing. I know it's obvious but your palms must face upward while holding the bar. You'll want to have your knee's slightly bent, which stops you rocking. If you're rocking, it gives you momentum to get the barbell up and that's only cheating yourself. No rocking, ok.

Z-BAR CURL: I like this bar more than the straight barbells only because it feels more comfortable on my wrists. Curling the straight bar strains my wrists. Holding the z-Bar prevents any wrist strain.

I only use the straight barbell when someone is already using the Z-Bar. But, if they're nearly finished, I'll wait.

CONCENTRATION CURL: This is done with 1 dumbbell and sitting on a padded seat. With my legs apart so that they make a 90 degrees angle, I can rest the back of the working arm against the inside of my knee.

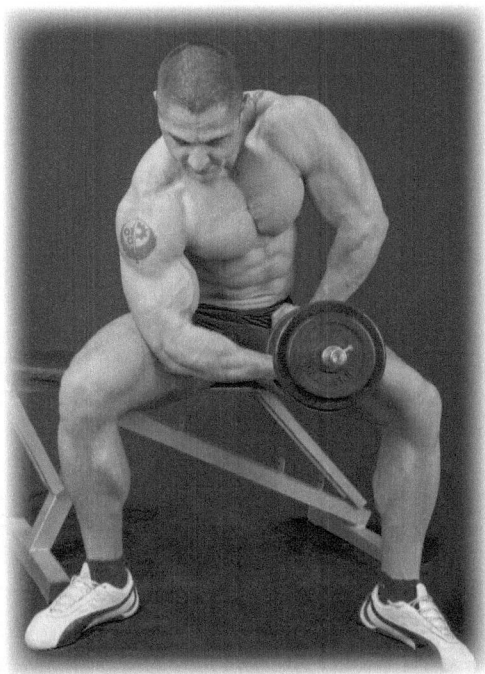

PULLEY CURL: Done using a short bar attached to a pulley which comes up from the ground. These are great because they keep constant tension on your bicep, throughout the whole movement. Like concentration curls, you will only use a light weight.

PREACHER CURLS: This is the barbell version of concentration curls. There is a special incline pad for this exercise, which can be used while standing or attached to a seated bench.

Holding the barbell, your triceps and elbows rest on the inclined pad. With your upper arms locked and unable to help swing the bar up, it's much harder than normal barbells or dumbbell curls which also means the weights you use are much lighter also.

FOREARM EXERCISES

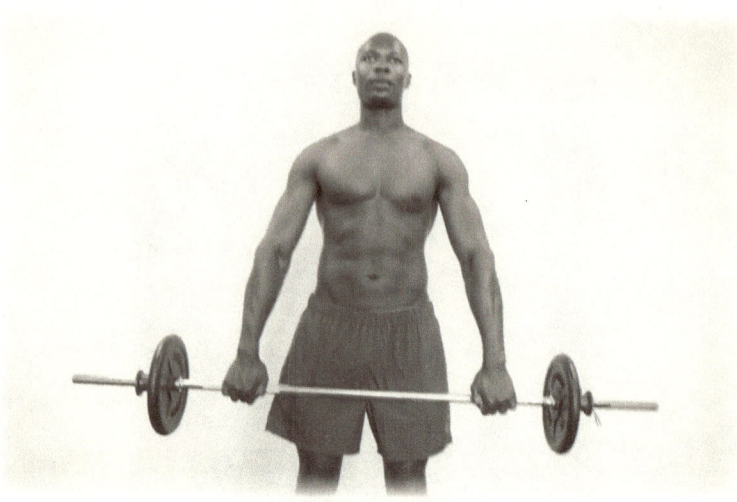

WRIST CURLS: For this exercise, you need a barbell and a flat bench to sit on. You'll sit on the bench with one leg on either side. Holding the barbell, you rest your forearms on the bench with your hands hanging over the edge of the bench. Grab the bar with palms facing up. You also need to grab the barbell in a close grip, say 6 to 8 inches apart.

The only movement is in your wrists. Raise and lower the barbell while your forearms sit on the padded bench. The reason you hang your hands and wrists over the edge of the bench is to give you a bigger range of movement.

REVERSE CURLS: You do this exercise with a barbell or Z-bar, in a standing position. Grab your bar overhand i.e, palms facing down. When you grab the bar, hold it with your elbows pushed firm into your side. Locking your elbows this way forces you to use your forearms only, and not cheat by swinging the bar up.

You must be careful not to swing the bar up. You raise it in a controlled manner. And, lower it with control. That is, don't just let gravity pull your arms down too quickly. Allowing gravity to influence your form will affect your results.

GRIP MACHINE: This is just a small machine with a rope attached to a weight. All you do is twisting a small bar with the rope attached, which winds the rope up as you twist it. As you twist the bar, the winding rope lifts the attached weight. It's a small machine that can be used next to a bench, so you're sitting as you use it.

Another type of similar machine has two small bars that you squeeze together. As you squeeze, it lifts an attached weight, for added resistance.

Either type is effective for building your forearms and a very strong handshake.

Well, that's my list of exercises in full.

WARM UP / WARM DOWN

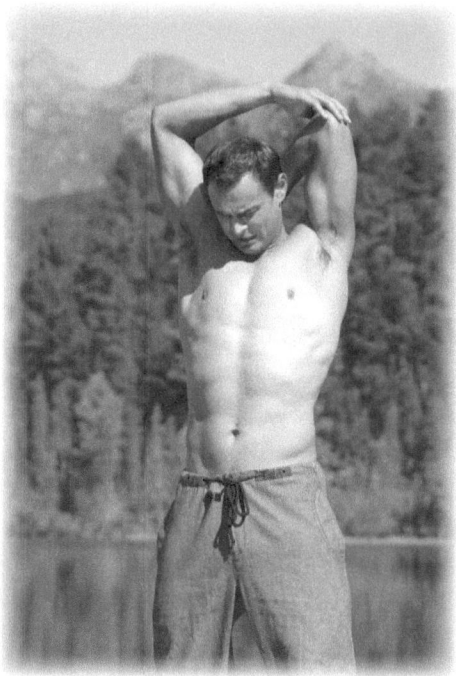

WARM UP: Every muscle must be warmed up before you get into its full swing. You can do this easily enough. Which ever exercise you start with for a particular muscle group; it will be used to warm up that muscle.

Take chest for example. I do bench press first. So my chest warm-up consists of two sets of lighter weights. The first one is pretty light and the second set is a little heavier.

You need to rep it out to 10 or 12 reps as well. Don't do the target 8 reps that you do for your counted sets. You're using a lighter weight so the extra reps are no problem.

By the time you've finished your bench press, your chest muscles are warmed up and ready for the other chest exercises. There are two points to remember here; if the other exercises are isolation exercises, you can jump straight into them. But, if they are compound exercises, you need to do another warm-up rep or two with that exercise.

Just to re-cap; Isolation exercises are usually light weights and hit just one muscle. Compound exercises are heavier and hit several muscles at the same time, during the exercise.

WARM DOWN: if you have the time, use an exercise bike or a treadmill for several minutes after you've finished your workout.

If you've got people to see or places to go and can't spare the time on the treadmill or bike, then some simple stretching will be enough to get you by. It's just to help with the blood flow and prevent some of the soreness that can occur.

Another thing I enjoy after a hard workout is a Whey Protein drink. Most gym's can whip one up in a few minutes. I don't take them after every workout, just as I feel like it.

PUTTING IT ALL TOGETHER

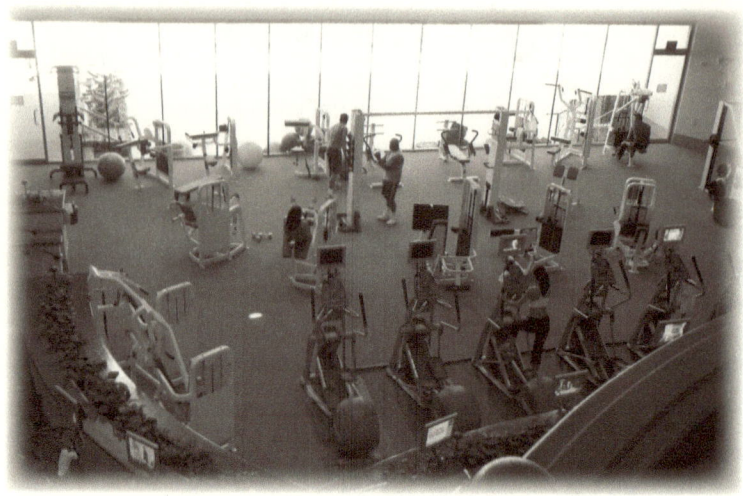

2 DAY SPLIT ROUTINE: This means dividing the muscles into groups. I find the most effective combinations as follows: Workout 1: Chest, Triceps, Shoulders and Abs. Workout 2: Legs, Back, Biceps and Forearms.

In earlier chapters, I talked about how some muscle groups can go with others in a workout. I also mentioned that some muscle groups shouldn't be trained with others. Each of the two workouts in this "2 Day Split Routine" follows my rules on which muscle groups go best together.

From the chapters on each muscle group which outline all the different exercises, you can add up all the exercises and see that Workout '1' has 24 exercises to choose from. And, that Workout '2' has 25 exercises to choose from, for the 2 Day Split Routine. The 5 Day Routine uses all the exercises, yep that's right, all of them. Owww!

The reason there are so many is to give you some variety for your 2 Day Split Routine. Each muscle will only need 3 to 5 exercises per training session (workout). Legs are the exceptions to this rule, because they have several areas to train (i.e, calves, quads & hamstrings). You should do at least 6 of the leg exercises to cover all the three parts of your legs.

Another point I need to mention is that some of the exercises need to be swapped around as you please while others must be done. In the workouts below, I've marked the exercises (#) that you must do. So I'm saying that if you're picking 3 to 5 exercises for any muscle, the exercises marked (#) must be included in your picks.

At this point, it would be good to go back to chapter (11), "How Many Reps and How Many Sets". Briefly, when you're just starting out or coming back from a break, doing 2 sets is plenty, for each muscle group. Build up slowly over several months to the 3 or 4 sets that you do with each exercise. Remember, warm-up sets aren't included in any count towards sets.

2 DAY SPLIT ROUTINE: WORKOUT—1

Shoulders:	BEHIND NECK PRESS (#) 2 warm-ups
	DUMBELL PRESS (#)
	UPRIGHT ROW
	BENT SIDE LATERALS
	SIDE LATERALS
Back:	DEAD LIFT (#) 2 warm-up sets
	LAT PULLDOWN (#)
	SEATED PULLEY ROW (#)
	CHINUPS (#)
	BENT ROW
	SHRUGS
	1-ARM ROW
Bicep:	BARBELL CURL (#) 2 warm-up sets
	DUMBELL CURL (#)
	Z-BAR CURL
	CONCENTRATION CURL

	PULLEY CURL
	PREACHER CURL
Abbs:	CRUNCHES 25 to 50 reps on all Abbs
	INCLINE SITUP
	LEG RAISE
	SITUP CHAIR
	PULLEY CRUNCH
	KNEE UPS

Note:

\#

\#

\#

2 DAY SPLIT: WORKOUT 2

Legs:	SQUATT (#) 2 warm-up sets
	INCLINE PRESS (#) 2 warm-ups also
	LEG EXTENSION (#)
	LEG CURL (#)
	STIFF LEG DEAD LIFT (#)
	STANDING CALVE Pick at least one
	SEATED CALVE
	TOE PRESS
Chest:	BENCH PRESS (#) 2 warm-up sets
	PECK DECK
	BENCH FLY

	INCLINE PRESS
	DUMBELL BENCH PRESS
	DUMBELL PULLOVER
	CABLE CROSSOVER
Triceps:	Z-BAR PRESS (#) 2 warm-up sets
	LAT MACHINE PUSHDOWN (#)
	1 ARM TRICEP PRESS
	CLOSE GRIP BENCH PRESS
	DUMBELL DIPS
	KICKBACKS
	PARALLEL BAR DIPS
Forearm:	WRIST CURL (#)
	REVERSE CURL
	GRIP MANCHINE

Note: Typically, you'll do the 2 day Split Routine 4 days per week. Say for example; Monday, Tuesday, Thursday and Friday. I have also used it 6 days per week but no longer than 6 months or a little longer.

Your body will be better off on the next workout which is very intense and gives your muscles the required rest time.

See the chart here showing the alternate workouts for the 4 or 6 days per week, 2 Days Split routine. Each workout (1 & 2) is done either 2 or 3 times each.

Mon	Tue	Wed	Thur	Fri	Sat	Sun
workout 1	workout 2	workout 1	workout 2	workout 1	workout 2	

You can see, over 4 or 6 days, you just alternate the two workouts.

2 DAY SPLIT—OPTION (Day on / Day off routine)

I have given you my 4 Day per Week version for the 2 Day Split Routine. But, I want to tell you about another option you have with this same workout. It is for those of you who are just starting out. Your muscles are going to be sore for weeks until you get used to doing the weight training.

A better option, for my new friends out there who are just starting, is to train 3 days per week, instead of 4.

You're still doing the same exercises, using the same good form to prevent injury and making fast gains in strength and muscle size. Your muscles will appreciate the extra day's rest each week. You should use it for 3 months at least.

As you know, you're breaking the muscle cells down in the gym and time out of the gym is when they grow back bigger and stronger, as they prepare for more of the same. That is why you never just keep training the same muscles every day. To keep breaking them down with no time for recovery and growth, will actually shrink you. See long distance runners for example, they are very lean after constant overloading.

Where as a sprinter may look like a bodybuilder due to the short intense loading with plenty of rest time.

The other option therefore is the **Day On Day Off** routine. See the chart below.

Mon	Tue	Wed	Thu	Fri	Sat	Sun
	workout 1		workout 2		workout 1	
Mon	Tue	Wed	Thu	Fri	Sat	Sun
workout 2		workout 1		workout 2		

Mon	Tue	Wed	Thu	Fri	Sat	Sun
	workout 1		workout 2		workout 1	
Mon	Tue	Wed	Thus	Fri	Sat	Sun
workout 2		workout 1		workout 2		

See over 14 days, you're doing each workout (1 & 2) 3 times each. The good thing about this spin on the Two Day Split is the extra rest you get before training a muscle group again. If you count the days in workout 1, you'll see that you get 3 to 5 days of rest. It's the same for workout 2.

5 DAY ROUTINE: This is the routine you want to graduate in. Each workout is done once a week. It takes five days to complete the whole routine which covers your whole body.

There's a very good reason for doing each body part only once per week. That's because the intensity is very high as you use all the advanced techniques; your body needs the rest.

It you trained with high intensity on any body part for more than once per week, you would get progressive overload and eventually have to stop training, due to severe fatigue.

You might be tempted to think you should skip the 2 day Split Routine, and just start on this routine. To put it into perspective, that would be like building the roof of your house at the ground level without the walls to support it.

Your body needs a foundation to work on. At-least 12 months of muscle growth; using the 2 Day Split system is the kind of foundation I'm talking about. If you haven't trained before, then even longer would be better. You really want to be pushing some serious weight.

If you read this book through several times so that you fully grasp all that it's offering, you'll train like me as if we are gym partners with the same knowledge, on the same course to getting the most out of our time spent training.

Over the years I've trained, there have been times when I had a long break for various reasons. I've never jumped straight into the 5 day routine after a long break.

I know enough not to do that. I hope you can appreciate what I'm trying to say.

With either system, you'll make massive gains. You won't outgrow the 5 Day Routine as you do the 2 Day Split. For example, Dead Lifts, Squats and Bench Press are good gauges for which system to use. When you're using one and a half times your body weight, it's a good time to switch to the 5 Day System. i.e; if you weigh 80kg, when you're using 120kg for dead lifts, squats and bench press, you should handle the intensity of the 5 day routine. You'd be lucky to get there in under a year, but it's no race either.

5 DAY ROUTINE

See day 1, 2, 3, 4 and 5

Day 1: Shoulders + Abbs

Shoulders:	BEHIND NECK PRESS	2 warm-up sets
	DUMBELL PRESS	do all exercises
	UPRIGHT ROW	4 sets of 8 reps on all
	BENT SIDE LATERALS	
	SIDE LATERALS	
Abs:	CRUNCHES	
	INCLINE SITUP	25 to 50 reps for all sets
	LEG RAISE	
	SITUP CHAIR	
	PULLY CRUNCH	
	KNEE UP'S	

Note:

#

#

#

Day 2: Bicep + Forearm 5

Biceps:	BARBELL CURL	2 warm-up sets
	DUMBELL CURL	do all exercises
	Z-BAR CURL	4 sets of 8 reps on all
	CONCENTRATION CURL	
	PULLEY CURL	
	PREACHER CURL	
Forearm:	WRIST CURL	
	REVERSE CURL	
	GRIP MACHINE	

Note:

#

#

#

Day 3: Chest + Triceps

Chest:	BENCH PRESS	2 warm-up sets
	PECK DECK	do all exercises
	BENCH FLY	4 sets of 8 reps on all
	INCLINE PRESS	
	DUMBELL BENCH PRESS	
	DUMBELL PULLOVER	
	CABLE CROSSOVER	
Tricep:	Z-BAR PRESS	
	DUMBELL DIPS	
	1-ARM TRICEP PRESS	
	LAT MACHINE PUSHDOWN	
	KICKBACKS	
	PARALLEL BAR DIPS	

Note:

\#

\#

\#

Day 4: Legs

Legs:	SQUATT	2 warm-up sets
	INCLINE PRESS	2 warm-up sets
	LEG EXTENSION	do all exercises
	LEG CURL	4 sets of 8 reps on all
	STIFF LEG DEAD LIFT	
	STANDING CALVE RAISE	
	SEATED CALVE RAISE	
	TOE PRESS	

Note:

#

#

#

Day 5: Back + Abbs

Back:	DEAD LIFT	2 warm-up sets
	LAT PULLDOWN	do all exercises
	SEATED PULLEY ROW	4 sets of 8 reps on back
	CHINUPS	4 sets of 25 to 50 on abbs
	BENT ROW	
	SHRUGS	
	1-ARM ROW	
Abbs:	CRUNCH	
	INCLINE SITUP	
	LEG RAISE	
	SITUP CHAIR	
	PULLEY CRUNCH	
	KNEE UP'S	

Note:

#

#

#

TRAIN WITHOUT INJURIES

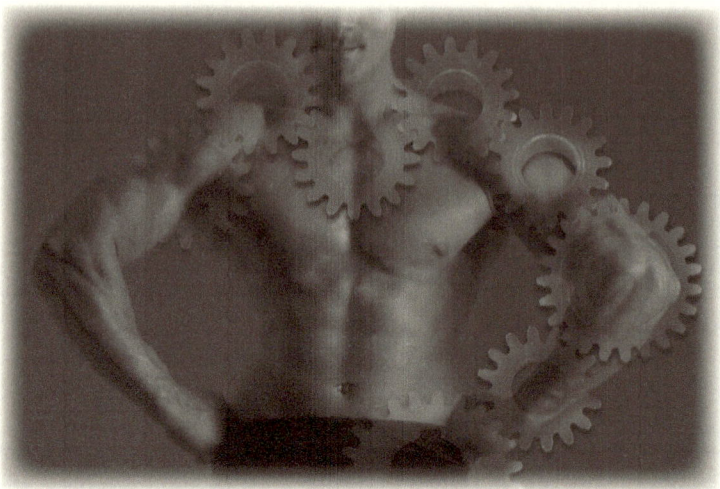

The last thing you want is an injury from training. It is worth mentioning because it is very frustrating to try to train around an injury.

The best way to avoid any injuries in the gym or at home for that matter is to adopt strict form right from the start. What does strict form mean?

In the gym, I am always aware of the position of my back. Never arch your back. When sitting up, or standing or leaning forward; you have to do it with a straight back.

You want to have your back supported at all times as well. I wear a weight belt on a lot of exercises such as squats, bent rows, seated pulley rows, upright rows, shoulder press, one arm rows and more. You get my point.

Another point on back support is the equipment in the gym. Padded seats for shoulder press will help you keep your back straight while you push big weights above your head. It makes good sense to lean against a padded seat every chance you can.

Going too heavy will surely give you a big chance of sustaining an injury. Big weights will come very quickly without being impatient and sacrificing on good form.

Another bi-product of too heavy and no form is jerking the weights up and down; a sure way to an injury. Just smooth and controlled movements win the race here. No sudden jerks in the hope of getting it off the ground or rack.

Swinging is another way I've seen people sustain their injuries. It looks awful and doesn't build muscles as fast as correct form with the right weights. Controlled movements up and down, not swinging, just to cheat and say you used a weight that is obviously too heavy.

I mentioned warming up and warming down. Cold muscles are at a higher risk of injury. It takes minutes to raise your body temperature on a bike or treadmill before you start your weights.

Stretching while you're sitting there waiting for your training partner to finish their set is a great idea. Stretch the muscle you're about to use. One stretch is better than none. Never stretch cold though. I shouldn't have to even write that.

Your equipment will help remove the risk of injuries. Your bare minimums are stable shoes and a weight belt. If I forgot my weight belt, I'd go home and get it. And I have done that.

Housekeeping in the gym: I've seen collars fall off a bar which lets the plates then fall off too. Toes and ankles seem to always be right in the way when that happens.

What happens if you do get an injury from training? You follow the P.R.I.C.E system.

P is for Protect yourself from further injury. Stop training.

R is for Rest your injury and take time out from training.

I is for Ice which needs to be applied for 20 minutes per hour for the first 72 hours.

C is for Compression which means apply a bandage if practical, or even a towel until you get home.

E is for Elevate, which means raise above your heart. You might have to lie down to do that.

You'll likely have 2 weeks off if you treat yourself with care. Do nothing and your recovery will be much longer. The ice treatment is so important if you expect a full recovery.

EATING FOR BODY BUILDING

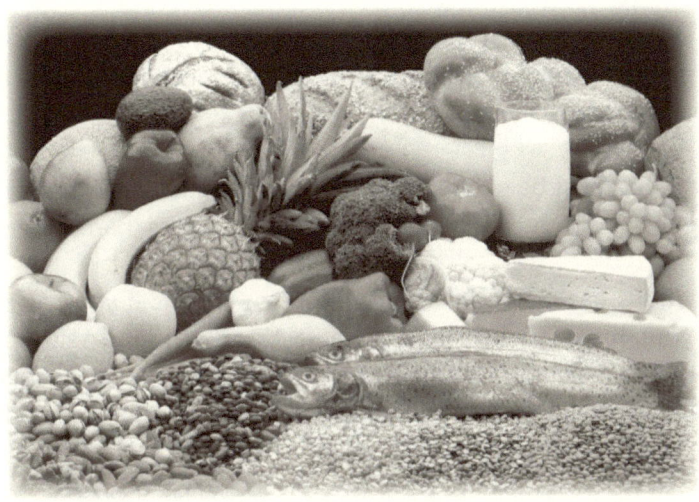

Cut fats, sugars and salt from your diet. No soft drinks, hot chips or potato chips, deep fried foods or lollies etc.

Complex carbohydrates are broken down into glucose more slowly than simple carbohydrates. More examples of these simple carbohydrates include anything made from sugar, or biscuits, jam, chocolate, cakes, lollies, liquorice, honey, softdrinks or tinned fruit.

Natural simple carbohydrates which are fine for weight loss include: apple, blackberry, black current, cherry, cranberry, grapefruit, kiwifruit, melon, orange, peach, pear, plum, raspberry, strawberry and pineapple.

Try to eat a breakfast each day. One that includes complex carbohydrates and some protein. How much protein per day? 1.50 grams per pound of your body weight.

It's been proven that regular small meals are best for balancing your blood sugar, plus it helps your metabolic rate. Any rise in your metabolic rate will help burn off excess fat.

Supplements with BCAA's are branched chained amino acids such as, leucine, isoleucine and valine. The minimum dose for these is 0.1 grams per pound of body weight.

Protein Tip: Try not to eat the same protein 2 days in a row. Supplement protein powders should be alternated daily too. Follow the protein plan for increased energy levels.

Carbohydrates must be eaten in every single meal to help the body absorb the protein. You should eat a little more carbohydrates than protein.

Small portions each day is best, having 5 to 7 meals if you can manage it. Split your breakfast into two, breakfast and morning tea. Split your lunch into two meals, lunch and afternoon tea. Have dinner or split in two with a late snack. The seventh meal can be your protein drink after your workout, when ever you do it.

The idea behind regular meals through the day is to reduce fat storage and raise your metabolism. Also to keep your blood sugar levels stable.

There is a wealth of information online as to what simple carbohydrates are. Just as a reminder here are a few examples refined sugar products, honey, fruit juices etc.

Also look up Complex Carbohydrates online. Some examples of these include oats, brown rice and sweet potato; Best eaten by 3.00pm daily.

Be aware that your body can crave sweet foods in the evenings when your serotonin levels are low. Avoid ice-creams, cookies, cakes etc.

Acceptable dietary fats include olive oil, salmon, tuna, nuts, seeds, avocados and peanut butter.

I always had a bottle of water in the gym with me too. You'll need to keep your muscles hydrated to avoid cramps. Half a Beroka or any other type of effervescent multi-B-vitamin tablet dissolved in the water will pep you up as good as those high priced products. I've tried them all, this is what I use.

www.ingramcontent.com/pod-product-compliance
Lightning Source LLC
Chambersburg PA
CBHW021545290526
45785CB00004BA/1521

* 9 7 8 1 4 5 2 5 0 9 1 9 8 *